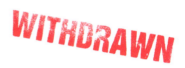

Sex Talk

Sex Talk

The Role of Communication in Intimate Relationships

CAREY M. NOLAND

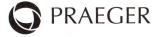 PRAEGER

AN IMPRINT OF ABC-CLIO, LLC
Santa Barbara, California • Denver, Colorado • Oxford, England

Library of Congress Cataloging-in-Publication Data
Noland, Carey M.
   Sex talk: the role of communication in intimate relationships / Carey M. Noland.
      p. cm.
   Includes bibliographical references and index.
   ISBN 978-0-313-37968-0 (alk. paper) — ISBN 978-0-313-37969-7 (ebook)
1. Sex.   2. Communication in sex.   3. Interpersonal communication.   4. Intimacy
(Psychology)   I. Title.
   HQ23.N65   2010
   306.7—dc22   2009051218

ISBN: 978-0-313-37968-0
EISBN: 978-0-313-37969-7

14   13   12   11   10   1   2   3   4   5

This book is also available on the World Wide Web as an eBook.
Visit www.abc-clio.com for details.

Praeger
An Imprint of ABC-CLIO, LLC

ABC-CLIO, LLC
130 Cremona Drive, P.O. Box 1911
Santa Barbara, California 93116-1911

This book is printed on acid-free paper ∞

Manufactured in the United States of America

To my mother, Donna Marie Noland, and husband, Hans Peter Schlecht, for all their love and support. Also, to Shelly Noland, a person generous of heart and kind in spirit.

Contents

CHAPTER 1

Why Is It Important to Learn about Communication about Sex? Some Straight Talk about Sex

I think sex is here to stay.

—*Groucho Marx*

I began my career as a health communication scholar and professor of interpersonal communication. In a close study of sexually transmitted infections and sexual education initiatives, I began to realize that interpersonal communication is sadly neglected in our society. While communication is one of the most important skills a person can have to ensure success in all aspects of his life, in general, we do not teach people how to communicate, let alone how to communicate in relationships and about sex. Communication is the way we connect with others and form and maintain personal relationships.

Connection with others is so essential to human beings that when a person is deprived of it for long periods of time, depression and self-doubt set in, and completing the essential tasks of daily life becomes difficult. Short of death, solitary confinement is the worse punishment that the U.S. penal system inflicts upon its most dangerous criminals. Numerous studies have confirmed that a close personal relationship with one other person is the most important factor in personal happiness, outranking job, money, and sex.[1] The desire for relationships is universal, and most people consider sex an integral component of a romantic relationship.

According to Paula Regan, a sexual attraction expert and professor at California State University, Los Angeles, "people believe that sexual desire is part and parcel of the state of being in love, assume that couples who desire each other sexually also are passionately in love, and report a similar association when reflecting on their own dating relationships."[2] Susan and Clyde Hendrick, both professors at Texas Tech University, developed a scale to measure participants' respect for their romantic partners. They found that relationship satisfaction, commitment, and self-disclosure were all linked and that those who had high levels of relationship satisfaction tended to have high levels of commitment and self-disclosure. In another study using the same survey, they measured how people viewed the link between love and sex in their romantic relationships. They found that most people thought that love was the most important thing in a relationship, that sex demonstrates love, that love comes before sex, and that sex generally declines as a relationship progresses. Both men and women viewed sexual intimacy as connected to relational intimacy, though their opinions about sex often diverged.[3] It is clear that most people believe sex is an essential aspect of love.

Sandra Metts and Brian Spitzberg, two communication scholars, note, "Sex may be one of life's greatest pleasures, but it is also a source of some of our thorniest interpersonal and social problems."[4] Another scholar notes, "It is a matter of some curiosity that a topic as salient and fascinating to so many of us as is sex should be one on which so little social scientific information is available."[5] Although we are fascinated with sex, we know embarrassingly little about the physical, emotional, and physiological issues associated with it. To bring much needed attention to these issues, this book focuses on sex in the United States and reviews the changing role of sex and sexuality in relationships, the value of learning more about sexual relationships from a communication perspective, and some of the of scholarly research that is available about sex, other than Kinsey and Masters and Johnson, the most well known studies done in the past 60 years.

In addition to reviewing and including the best and most up-to-date research from interpersonal communication, research on sex is also a main component of this book. In the 1980s people in the United States suddenly became more interested in the study of sexual relationships due to growing awareness of the role of sex in the spread of disease. The HIV/AIDS epidemic officially began on June 5, 1981, when the Centers for Disease Control and Prevention (CDC) issued a warning about a rare form of pneumonia.[6] With the advent of the HIV/AIDS epidemic, there has been an increase in the value of research about sexual knowledge, attitudes, and practices. Yet today, we have more HIV seropositive people than ever before. There were 1.1 million people in 2006 in the United States who were estimated to be living with HIV, and there are approximately 56,000 new cases annually.[7] As such, there has been a significant increase in grant money to study sexual relationships, and numerous publication outlets, such as academic journals, have begun to disseminate research on the topic of sexuality.

Global definitions of sexual health by the United Nations, the U.S. surgeon general, and a host of sex researchers focus on a more positive approach to sexual health than limiting it to definitions of disease and a source of social problems:

> Sexual health requires a respectful approach to sexual relationships, and that these relationships should be free of coercion, and present the possibility of pleasurable, safe experiences. According to these individuals and organizations, sexually healthy adults should take pleasure and pride in their bodies, and should be able to communicate honestly and openly with their partners. They should have a sense of their own sexual values and be relatively free of anxiety over their own sexuality and that of others. Finally, sexually healthy persons should have the ability to form interdependent and rewarding relationships.[8]

Notice the emphasis on communication and relationships. Representatives of major government institutions recognize the importance of both for sexual health.

A major goal of this book is to help people become competent communicators, especially in the area of sex. Being able to talk about sex with an openness and honesty will bring respect, peace of mind, and an understanding of communication breakdowns that occur around sexual topics. Good communication will improve the quality of our sexual relationships, monogamous and otherwise. Part of becoming a competent communicator involves raising individuals' level of consciousness about communication with partners because consciousness is necessary for communicating.

A competent communicator is someone who is effective and able to achieve her desired goal and someone who meets the expected rules or expectations for the communication context. Additionally, competent communicators possess an anticipatory mind-set. This means that they can anticipate the implications of their actions (for both parties) and foresee any obstacle that might impede the achievement of their goals. Therefore competent communicators will adjust their goals and plans in light of situational, relational, and/or cultural circumstances.[9] Specific competencies include verbal and nonverbal responsiveness, the ability to begin and sustain interesting conversations, the ability to self-disclose, the ability to provide emotional support, and the ability to manage conflict. Communication competence becomes especially important during adolescence, when creating and maintaining meaningful relationships outside the family becomes increasingly important because individuals generally desire to access and engage peers.

The quality of our sex lives is inextricably linked to the quality of our personal relationships and how well we receive and deliver our sexual messages. Talking about sex with a variety of different people in our lives, including our sexual partners, family members, and medical professionals, is vital to our becoming full and lively human beings. The truth is that establishing and maintaining not only interpersonal relationships, but also a good sex life, is hard work. The high American divorce rates strongly indicate that a majority of people have a difficult time with relationships, and specifically with sexual relationships. In a recent research report, more couples listed communication issues as their main relationship problem—more so than money problems or child-rearing issues.[10]

Sexual problems rank among the top three problems in the majority of studies on newly married couples.[11] When couples were interviewed later in their relationships, the sex problems had not diminished; rather, they just talked about them less often. It is safe to assume that people decide to live with sexual problems and not talk about them. Even people who reported being in happy marriages had sexual problems. One study found that approximately 80 percent of participants reported being in happy marriages, but 90 percent of these same people reported sexual problems in their happy marriages.[12] Can we also assume that people can be happy, yet in sexually unsatisfying marriages? Other research shows that sexual frequency (or infrequency) does not lead to the dissolution of relationships; however, poor sexual quality does. In other words, sexual satisfaction is more closely tied to quality, and a lack of quality leads to relationship dissolution.

Since the large majority of sexually active adults are married or cohabiting, the vast majority of instances of sexual intercourse at any given time in the nation will occur between married or cohabiting partners. In these cases, the partner has been chosen not exclusively or even primarily for sexual potential. Sex is only one of the relevant factors influencing marital choice. The partner is, typically, a resident partner, a financial partner, a social partner, a confidant and friend, and a coparent of one's children as well as a sex partner. The choice of a spouse or long-term partner reflects these several dimensions of the relationship, and sexual compatibility is not the only, or necessarily the most important, factor. This means that as we reflect on the positives of our own sexual experience with our primary partners, the quality of the overall relationship is assessed, not just the quality of the sexual relationship.[13] However, as AnnaMaria Giraldi, editor of the *Journal of Sex Medicine*, recently outlined in an editorial, the role of sex has dramatically changed over the years.[14]

Historically, couples had sex to procreate. Couples stayed together for a variety of reasons, including religious beliefs, the economic dependence of women on male partners, other family obligations, and the stigma against multiple sexual partners as well as the inherent trust assumed in a marital commitment. Sexual satisfaction was rarely a topic many couples discussed, and it was even rarer that someone would end a marriage because of the quality of his sex life. However, as Giraldi argues, times have changed, noting that we can have children without sex and sex without having children. The focus of sex has shifted from procreation to recreation, and people in the United States have particularly high expectations for sex. For most Americans, sex is now directly related to quality-of-life issues, and given the high numbers of people with sexually transmitted infections, having safe sex is of the utmost concern.

The role of commitment and relationships regarding sex has also significantly shifted from past generations. Before, there were basically two socially acceptable options for people: either you were married and had sex or you were single (or widowed) and you were not supposed to have sex. For the majority of Americans, there was only one option for sex: to be in a fully committed, married relationship. Now we have an entirely different continuum of sex activity, ranging from sex without commitment in terms of hooking up; sex in a casual relationship in a friends-with-benefits relationship; sex between people who are in a committed dating relationship; sex between people who cohabitate and choose not to get married; and sex between those who are in committed, married relationships. How we talk about sex greatly depends on the type of sexual relationship, as each kind of sexual activity requires different approaches and skills. By understanding the differences between these kinds of relationships, one can tailor one's understanding of the role of communication in that situation, the boundaries associated with each kind of situation, and the costs and benefits of each kind of relationship.

Recent surveys show that many Americans are living in sexless marriages.[15] Experts define a sexless marriage as making love fewer than

10 times per year. Estimates indicate that 40 million people are living in sexless marriages, and it is often the man who refuses sex—or is at least as likely as the woman to decline sexual advances. Now, if both people in the marriage are satisfied with a sexless marriage, then there is not a great problem. However, most people would prefer to have a robust sex life.

What does a robust sex life mean? How much sex are typical Americans having? Married couples say they have sex 68.5 times a year, or slightly more than once a week, according to a 2002 study by the National Opinion Research Center at the University of Chicago, and the numbers had not changed much over the previous 10 years.[16] According to the survey, people who are married only have 6.9 more sexual encounters a year than people who have never been married (single people). Estimates of sexual frequency vary according to different surveys. For example, according to a 2003 Durex survey of approximately 3,000 people in the United States, couples living together report having sex 146 times per year, while married couples report making love 98 times per year. Single people report that they have sex around 49 times a year.

In 2003, a world survey was conducted to see what men and women had to say about the ideal number of sexual partners they would like to have in one month.[17] In North America, 23 percent of men surveyed said more than one, whereas only 3 percent of women said more than one. To some extent, this does confirm the assumption that men prefer more sexual variety than women, but it is not to the extent that many would assume. Less than one in four men would like more than one partner, which is a relatively small number of people. When broken down by cultural region of the world, South America had the highest percentages, with 35 percent of men and 6.1 percent of women indicating that they would want more than one sexual partner next month. Other regions, including Western Europe, where approximately 22.6 percent of men and 5.5 percent of women; Eastern Europe, with 31.7 percent of men and 7.1 percent of women; Southern Europe, with 31 percent of men and 6 percent of women; the Middle East, with 33.1 percent of men and 5.9 percent of women; Africa, with 18.2 percent of men and 4.2 percent of women; Oceania, with 23.3 percent of men and 5.8 percent of women; South/Southeast Asia, with 32.4 percent of men and 6.4 percent of women; and East Asia, with 17.9 percent of men and 2.6 percent of women, reported that they wanted more than one sexual partner. When the question of whether a person wanted more than one partner in the next month was specifically asked to those who indicated that they were pursuing short-term sexual relationships, 50 percent of the men said yes, whereas only 20 percent of the women said yes. This means that women are likely to want fewer partners and even exclusivity, even in short-term sexual encounters. Overall, the majority of people around the world would clearly prefer one sexual partner.

INTERPERSONAL COMMUNICATION AND SEX TALK

Interpersonal communication scholars view sexual communication as a complex, dynamic process, in which "sexual partners are *active participants*, who each have their own set of *goals* and the ability to choose *strategies* to maximize goal achievement."[18] Furthermore, people have different goals during sex. People report that goals during sex include "fulfilling sexual desire, maintaining a positive self-image, pleasing their partner, strengthening the relationship, relieving tension, and preserving health."[19] Sometimes these goals could conflict: if a person is having sex to please her partner but wants to preserve her health, it may be difficult if a partner refuses to use a condom. Since sex is overwhelmingly an activity involving two people, the sexual practices that are undertaken are jointly experienced, but the two people may have quite different assessments of the sexual act and probably experience the same sexual event in very different ways. If you think about it, sex occurs in a "nonshared environment," even for the two individuals involved. This means that two people who have sex together do not experience the same sexual act the same way. Both partners may not enjoy the same activity. Both cannot get pregnant. Both may not wish to be engaged in sex at the same time and in the same circumstances. It is likely that each person will walk away from a sexual interaction with different interpretations of the same event. As a result, the importance of meaningful communication cannot be overstated.

Some people may believe that perhaps sex is so instinctive, so primal, that no lessons are needed and no information is required. We have, after all, seemed to figure out how to have babies, increase the population, and get on with having pretty good sex lives without academic research to guide us. However, the sexual choices that we make, both privately and collectively, matter.

Personal decisions that comprise our sexual choices have effects and ramifications that range from the personal to the public. Results can range from getting a sexually transmitted infection that cannot be cured to a pregnancy that inadvertently creates a new life with a lifetime bond and mutual obligations between parent and child. Similarly, the effect on the community can be substantial, ranging from decisions about any of the sexual behaviors or practices that involve sexually transmitted infections to the problems of teenage childbearing, the dependence on welfare of single teenage mothers, access to and funding of abortion, the promotion of birth control and disease prevention, rape, sexual harassment, pornography, nudity, infidelity, and on and on. Topics relating to sexual behavior are among the most explosive and divisive in many of our communities. Better information may not solve these complex problems, but information can improve the sexual choices that we make, both privately and collectively, and decrease consequences, both privately and collectively.[20]

COMMUNICATION ABOUT SEX AND RELATIONSHIPS IS IMPORTANT

There are many important reasons to learn about sex and communication—to study the communication within sexual relationships. Where do we first learn about sexual relationships? For most of us, it is at home and at school. One might imagine that sex education programs in school are taking care of relationship issues involved with sex, yet research shows that this is not the case. In a study of Canadian high school students who had received extensive sex education throughout their formal schooling, respondents reported that their friends, family, and forms of popular culture were their main sources of information about sexual health and that "the type of information received from these sources (feelings, decisions, and experiences) was not available through formal channels. Students thought that sex education classes offered the technical information. . . . Sex education classes did not provide them with information they found useful."[21] When asked what was missing, the people in the study reported such things as the emotional aspects of sexuality, relationship issues, communication with partners, and gender differences. In essence, students felt that their education about sex and reproduction was adequate, whereas their education about communication, relationships, and sex was not. It is little wonder that these students crave such knowledge since the reality is that most people find it difficult to talk about sex within relationships. Whereas much of public health education about sex focuses on developing practices of safer sex and basic reproduction, this information ignores the reality of our personal relationships. Communication scholars have long studied topics that are considered off limits for many couples. There are a number of taboo topics in close relationships, including the state of the relationship, extrarelational activity, relationship norms, prior relationships, conflict-generating topics, self-disclosures perceived as unpleasant to discuss, and safe sex.[22]

The study of sexuality from a communication perspective thus introduces and increases our understanding of how the nature and context of relationships create and influence our communication about sex. The communication perspective also introduces something more that public health education does not or often has not. Considerable research shows that while some public health interventions have, to their credit, increased knowledge and use of safer sex practices and slightly lessened some of the unwanted health consequences of human sexual activity, many people still do not enact protective behaviors despite their knowledge about safer sex practices. The truth is that most Americans know about the effectiveness of abstinence, monogamy, and consistent condom use and yet still engage in unprotected or dangerous sexual activities. Therefore we must admit that the view of humans and sex encompasses the idea that much more than knowledge is involved. On many levels we know what to do and why; we just do not do it. This book explains why we do not and how we can overcome many of the barriers that prevent us from doing the right thing by using communication techniques.

There are many reasons why we do not talk about sex and why many of us are uninformed about sexual issues. First, because sex is intimate, we are reluctant to ask for advice about the topic or even signal to trusted friends or family members that we might in fact need such advice. Because sex is such a private and personal act, less information, experience, and knowledge about this domain of life is shared than as compared to most others. We do not readily share our knowledge of sex, nor is our knowledge necessarily of interest to our family members and friends since our own experience is partner-specific. While there are many how-to books, articles, videos, and gurus offering advice about sex, that advice is typically anecdotal, entertainment-oriented, focused on the unusual or the bizarre, and typically not very useful.[23] Because of the reluctance to discuss sexual behavior, it is difficult to discern high-quality advice from bad advice. As Robert Michael, sex policy researcher, notes, "Few of us have ever been directly instructed in sexual behavior by a trusted and caring family member or by a loved one who was not actually a sex partner; few of us have ever observed other couples having sex. The stylized and scripted events of popular films, television shows, and novels certainly do not offer much useful information in this regard."[24] In actuality, we have very few quality sources from which to learn about sexual relationships.

WHO ARE PEOPLE TALKING TO ABOUT SEX?

It should be easy to talk about sex. You do not need a medical degree to know how sex works. In fact, most people know that it is important to talk about sex for many reasons, and they even have a good idea of what to say. But research shows that it is actually very difficult for people to talk about sex in meaningful ways with the people who are most important to them. Almost all of our sex education and public service announcements focus on disease prevention and largely ignore the reality of our personal relationships. People do not feel comfortable and/ or truthful when talking about sex with sexual partners,[25] family members,[26] and medical professionals.[27] One alarming set of research clearly documents that young people, in particular, are notoriously reluctant to discuss safer sex with their romantic partners.[28] The one exception with whom people report high levels of comfort speaking about sex is with friends—primarily female friends.[29] In a large-scale longitudinal survey over 17 years of over 6,000 students, researchers consistently found that college students reported speaking about sex with peers more than parents or any other group of people.[30] Over time, researchers found an increase in the amount of communication about sex with professionals and peers. First-year college students talk to their friends more than their mothers about sex, and the frequency of communication about sex was correlated with frequency of sexual activity.[31] In communication with male friends, males reported that almost all the conversations were in a joking manner and described the content of their sex talk as revolving around things such as how to get a girl, what they wanted to do with women, and what they liked and disliked about their partners, especially past partners. Interestingly, with women, it is very similar: most women joked about sex but spoke more directly about their sexual likes and dislikes and about their partners' sexual performances. However, most people do not have sex with their friends, so there is limited usefulness in sex talk with friends. Friends are usually not medical experts on sexual issues and rarely have significantly more knowledge than one another. It would be helpful if people also talked to their actual sex partners and even medical providers about their sexual activities.

Much of the current literature about who people talk to about sex concludes that people do not have the communication skills to engage in health-protective sexual communication. Part of this is due to our sexual education. There are major deficiencies in both formal and informal sexuality education.[32] Much current North American research supports these conclusions: skill-based intervention programs are not equipping people, particularly young women, with the necessary communication skills to engage in protective sexual behaviors.

INFLUENCES ON RESEARCH ABOUT SEX AND COMMUNICATION ABOUT SEX

We do not know much about human sexuality for many reasons. For many decades it has been difficult to collect research about the different aspects of sex because it was considered a taboo topic. Realistically, it is difficult to collect data on sexual attitudes, behaviors, and practices. Also, because sex is natural, we all assumed that we should naturally know how to do it, how to talk about it, and how to solve problems associated with it. Furthermore, some who believe that sex research should not be undertaken have successfully influenced government policy and discouraged such research. Consequently, little research has been conducted and little knowledge accumulated about sexual behavior until the past decade.

It is a matter of some curiosity that a topic as salient and fascinating to so many of us as is sex should be one on which so little social scientific information is available. There is, to be sure, a lot of media exposure given to sex, but most of that is either pure entertainment, a sales vehicle, or part of some political agenda. However, for several decades now, a small number of social science researchers have undertaken ordinary, useful scientific research on aspects of sexual behavior. While that work has been fruitful, it has remained peripheral.

Many contextual and situational features may influence the discussion of sexual practices between partners. Within the context of places or arenas of discussion like the family or the school, the discussion of sexual practices may create a series of potential problems. Schools typically are not going to encourage adolescents to think about different ways to handle sexual interactions. Many parents, as well as schools, do not want to be viewed as encouraging sexual interaction. Many schools fear a negative reaction from the public more than the potential for adolescents' infection with sexually transmitted infections (STIs) or teen pregnancy.[33]

As discussed, one of the problems with sex education materials available is their emphasis on safer sex and sexual health. Yet many of these educational units do not work within the reality of our relationships. We must consider that reality both in terms of relationship development issues and contextual factors that influence our communication. For example, research about relationship development clearly shows that "couples frequently begin having sex before they are comfortable talking about intimate emotional issues. Cultural norms and gender inequality also inhibit honest discussion of safer sex."[34] "Despite the effectiveness of consistent and careful condom use, many sexually active Americans are still engaging in unprotected sexual activities."[35] Likewise, many people know they should talk about sex with important people in their lives. For example, parents know they should talk to their adolescent children about sex, yet few adults and children actually know how to do this or want to do this. In a study I conducted about sex, I asked participants what people should do to stop the spread of STIs and decrease unplanned pregnancies. Every person in the interview offered numerous suggestions about what could be done, and almost every one of the people said, "It all starts at home. Parents need to talk to their children about sex more." I responded to each person with the following questions. I asked the people who had children, "Do you want to talk to your children more about sex?" Every person answered no. I asked the younger participants, "Do you want to talk to your parents more about sex?" Every person responded the same way: no. People realize the importance of talking about sex; they just do not want to *personally* talk about it with their family members.

Much of our communication around sex—although often thought to be very private—carries with it consequences that extend to the relationship as a whole and to society in general. In the face of some of the more public of these consequences (e.g., unwanted or unplanned pregnancies, transmission of STIs, the pandemic of AIDS, sexual coercion), both political and medical entities have taken a great interest in the consequences of private sexual relationships. For the most part, sex surfaces as a subject of inquiry when it costs money: when medical expenses are incurred, when welfare checks are written to single mothers, when police protection is required in cases of sexual abuse, or when the explicit sale of sex is a focus of a vice squad raid, for example.

However, political, economic, and medical entities are not best positioned to study the mediating environment of sex, which is human communication. As a result, much of the research that has been done to understand, intercede, and control the consequences of human sexual relationships has been focused on information and education, not communication per se, and not on the relational aspect of sex. Indeed, much of the research that has been done about sex has been done in the face of negative consequences, problematizing sex instead of striving to understand the possibilities of our sexual relationships. After all, the driving forces for most research on sexuality have been concerns related to HIV/AIDS and other STIs, women's and men's reproductive health, contraceptive use, erectile dysfunction, and related issues.

The result is that "sexuality is negatively viewed as the source of problems and disease rather than an integral part of human development and health."[36] To rectify this situation, it is argued that "the usefulness of this research should not be limited to a problem-solving approach, even though sexuality research can provide crucial information and provide a greater understanding of such challenges as teenage pregnancy, HIV/AIDS, and sexual coercion."[37] Thus we need to explore communication around sex in relationships without presuming any negative consequences of sex itself: sexual harassment, coercion, and disease. More recently, "sexual communication has been identified as one of the key components in understanding the interpersonal interactions that facilitate or impede sexual health protective behaviors."[38] More and more medical researchers are focusing on the interpersonal aspects of human sexuality in their research.

Much of the current self-help literature or information about sex from sex therapists focuses on the exciting but atypical aspects of sex. This book focuses on the aspects of sex that are more typical than atypical. Rather than problematizing sex, I place it in a context of everyday realities because sex is part of the every day. The nature of everyday relationships, with all their tedium and repetitious boredom, has been allowed to be represented in books as abnormal and something to be avoided, particularly when it comes to sex. However, these portrayals essentially lead to the endorsement of the caricature that relationships are composed of all (and only) those exciting and dramatic or bizarre things to which both media and researchers have so far given their attention—as if everyday life were like the news headlines, which it is not. The goal of this book is to help you make sex talk a normal, comfortable part of your life so you can address this important aspect of life.

Indeed, if we characterize sexual talk as something dramatic and exotic, it places too much stress on the event and gives it the appearance of being atypical. For example, think about "the talk"—the sex talk between parents and adolescents. There is a great deal of buildup around this singular moment: anxieties, embarrassment, dread . . . the list goes on. However, there are significant problems with "the talk." First, "the talk" usually does not work because there is not a perfect moment to sit down and have it. What age is best? Is the discussion prompted by questions? Do the adolescents even understand what they are asking? What is the appropriate level of maturity necessary for the talk? What is occurring in sexual education classes at school? What are the child's friends talking about? Parents try to plan for the perfect moment, but there is no perfect moment; rather, it is important to gather information gradually and have an ongoing conversation with your adolescents so that you can adjust topic information and level of detail based on the information you have gathered from previous talks. Normally, "the talk" is portrayed as the child sitting down to listen to a lecture from the parent. However, these talks should not be one way; rather, they should be transactional, where both parties have equal opportunities to participate. You cannot have "the talk" just once and consider it done; it needs to be an ongoing conversation. This is one example of the type of information about sex talk that will be covered in this book. It is important to keep in mind that most people have formed their own opinions about sex and use their personal experiences to weigh research and public information about sex when it is presented to them in different forms.

COMMUNICATION IS ESSENTIAL

Communication in general is an exceedingly practical art. Understanding and applying theories of interpersonal communication and research to your talks about sex and your relationships in general will be extremely helpful. The more you know about communication, the more insight and knowledge you will gain about what works in sex talk and what does not. The skills you learn regarding sex talk will be applicable to other parts of your life, particularly those that include topics that fall under the umbrella of difficult conversations. Theories, research, and skills are presented in this book together and will help you as we progress through the elements of communication about sex, the ways nonverbal and verbal messages operate in sexual relationships, and the ways sexual relationships are developed and maintained and even repaired.

Most people have their own theories about how to talk about sex. But with the help of research completed by communication scholars, medical professionals, psychologists, sociologists, and anthropologists, people have the opportunity to become better equipped to communicate in a manner that is more valid, reliable, and comprehensive.

Communication itself is a process and plays an important role in our lives. Through interpersonal communication, we try to meet our social and psychological needs. We need to interact with other people, and through this interaction, we develop a sense of self and learn how other people see us. It is essential to recognize that interpersonal communication is learned. If your family believed it was rude to interrupt people, then you probably do not interrupt people. If it was necessary to yell and interrupt people to be heard in your family, then you learned to yell and interrupt people. If your teachers told you to look them in the eye when they were talking to you, then you look people in the eye when talking to them to show respect. If you went to a school where teachers said things like "don't be eyeballing me when I am talking to you," you learned that it was respectful to have a downcast glance when showing respect. The manner in which we communicate is learned behavior. Learning is a continual process, however, and you can apply what you learn from this book to your life and improve your interpersonal skills.

As people investigate all that is involved in communication about sex in relationships, they try to understand the dynamics of relationships that blend into relationship realities to make communication about sex possible and impossible, likely or less likely, timely or untimely, helpful or hurtful within romantic relationships. When the words *communication about sex* are used, this means any communication about sex, verbal or nonverbal, thus including communicative acts such as expression of desire, discussion of sexual likes and dislikes, disclosure of sexual history and experiences, verbal and nonverbal expressions of intimacy, communication and metacommunication involving the sexual aspects of the overall romantic relationship, building of sexual and relational intimacy, and so on. Many such communicative acts fall under the relationship dimension of self-disclosure, something that is imperative for relationship development and maintenance.

CONCLUSION

Sex plays an important role in our lives. Research in human sexuality has found that engaging in sexual activity is good for the body.[39] Those benefits are both physical and psychological. Physical benefits (from arousal and orgasm) include improvements to the respiratory, immune, circulatory, and cardiovascular systems. Psychological benefits include decreased stress, depression, and anxiety and increased levels of vitality. More specifically, researchers have identified that sexual activity has at least six potential outcomes: physical pleasure; emotional satisfaction; intimate bonding with one's partner that may promote love; reputation or peer judgment; the probability of pregnancy; and the probability of transmission of disease. Generally, people have sex to gain the first two or three of these products, and occasionally the fourth or fifth, but never the sixth.[40]

In Western culture, just how important is sex? Interpersonal relationship experts Susan Sprecher and Kathleen McKinney show that general relationship satisfaction and love are highly correlated to sexual satisfaction.[41] Dr. Charles Marwick reported the results of an opinion poll of 500 people that found that 91 percent of married men ranked a satisfying sex life as important, as did 84 percent of married women. These results highlight that as humans, the quality of our sex life is linked to our health, happiness, and sense of wellness. Conversely, an unsatisfactory sex life is highly problematic: over 90 percent of those polled by Dr. Marwick believed that sexual problems lead to depression, emotional distress, extramarital affairs, and the breakup of marriages. Unsatisfactory sex can (and does) lead to the dissolution of commitment. I will never be so simplistic to suggest that more communication about sex in relationships guarantees better sex and therefore better relationships and stronger commitment, but I do claim that we should understand more about the everyday communication about sex that we have within our relational realities, and part of those relational realities relates commitment to sex.

Although it is difficult to establish a direct cause-effect link between happiness and sexual satisfaction, there have been some recent studies that show strong positive associations between emotional well-being and sexual satisfaction, particularly in women. A recent Australian study showed a link between positive mood scores and sexual satisfaction in healthy, nondysfunctional women.[42] Likewise, there are numerous studies that show a link between sexual dysfunction and lower quality-of-life scores and weak well-being assessments.[43] Increasingly in society, the public demand for information about sex is greater than ever, and as a society, we talk more and more about sex. Due to the Internet and other media sources, the subject of sex and sexuality is more accessible today to the mainstream public than it has ever been before in history.

NOTES

1. Christiane Laroche and Gaston-Rene de Grace, "Factors of Satisfaction Associated with Happiness in Adults," *Canadian Journal of Counselling* 31, no. 4 (1997).

2. Paula Regan, "Sex and the Attraction Process: Lessons from Science (and Shakespeare) on Lust, Love, Chastity, and Fidelity," in *The Handbook of Sexuality in Close Relationships*, ed. John Harvey, Amy Wenzel, and Susan Sprecher (Mahwah, NJ: Lawrence Erlbaum Associates, 2004), 115.

3. Susan Sprecher and Kathleen McKinney, *Sexuality* (Newbury Park, CA: Sage, 1993).

4. Sandra Metts and Brian Spitzberg, "Sexual Communication in Interpersonal Contexts: A Script-Based Approach," in *Communication Yearbook*, ed. Brant Burleson (Mahwah, NJ: Lawrence Erlbaum Associates, 1996), 49.

5. Robert Michael, "Private Sex and Public Policy," in *Sex, Love, and Health in America: Private Choices and Public Policies*, ed. Edward Laumann and Robert Michael (Chicago: University of Chicago Press, 2000), 487.

6. Centers for Disease Control and Prevention, "Pneumocystis Pneumonia—Los Angeles," *Mortality and Morbidity Weekly Report 1981* (Atlanta, GA: Centers for Disease Control and Prevention, 1981), 30.

7. Centers for Disease Control and Prevention, "HIV/AIDS Surveillance Report: Cases of HIV Infection and AIDS in the United States, 2005," Centers for Disease Control and Prevention, http://www.cdc.gov/hiv/stats/2005Surveil lanceReport.pdf.

8. Allison S. Caruthers, "'Hookups' and 'Friends with Benefits': Nonrelational Sexual Encounters as Contexts of Women's Normative Sexual Development" (UMI Microform 3192595, ProQuest Information & Learning, 2006), 29.

9. Joy Koesten, "Family Communication Patterns, Sex of Subject, and Communication Competence," *Communication Monographs* 71 (2004).

10. National Communication Association, *How Americans Communicate* (Washington, DC: National Communication Association, 2009).

11. Philip Blumstein and Pepper Schwartz, *American Couples: Money, Work, Sex* (New York: Morrow, 1983).

12. Jonathan Freedman, *Happy People: What Happiness Is, Who Has It and Why* (New York: Ballantine, 1978).

13. Michael, "Private Sex and Public Policy," 467.

14. AnnaMaria Giraldi, "Sex Is Here to Stay," *Journal of Sex Medicine* 5, no. 2737–2739 (2008).

15. Bob Berkowitz and Susan Yaeger-Berkowitz, *He's Just Not up for It Anymore: Why Men Stop Having Sex and What You Can Do about It* (New York: HarperCollins, 2007).

16. National Opinion Research Center at the University of Chicago, *GSS Report*, ed. University of Chicago (Chicago: University of Chicago, 2003).

17. David Schmitt, "Short and Long Term Mating Strategies: Additional Evolutionary Systems Relevant to Adolescent Sexuality," in *Romance and Sex in Adolescence and Emerging Adulthood: Risks and Opportunities*, ed. Ann C. Crouter and Alan Booth (Mahwah NJ: Lawrence Erlbaum Associates, 2006), 43.

18. David Dryden Henningsen, Mary Lynn Miller Henningsen, and Kathleen S. Valde, "Gender Differences in Perceptions of Women's Sexual Interest during Cross-Sex Interactions: An Application and Extension of Cognitive Valence Theory," *Sex Roles* 54, no. 11 (2006): 87.

19. Richard Perloff, *Persuading People to Have Safer Sex: Applications of Social Science to the AIDS Crisis* (Mahwah, NJ: Lawrence Erlbaum Associates, 2001), 39.

20. Michael, "Private Sex and Public Policy," 467.

21. A. DiCenso, V. W. Borthwick, C. A. Busca, C. Creatura, J. A. Holmes, W. F. Kalagian, and B. M. Partington, "Completing the Picture: Adolescents Talk about What's Missing in Sexual Health Services," *Canadian Journal of Public Health* 92, no. 1 (2001): 36.

22. Leslie A. Baxter and William W. Wilmot, "Secret Tests: Social Strategies for Acquiring Information about the State of the Relationship," *Human Communication Research* 11 (1984). Perloff, *Persuading People*, 39.

23. Michael, "Private Sex and Public Policy."

24. Ibid., 489.

25. Leanne K. Knobloch and Katy E. Carpenter-Theune, "Topic Avoidance in Developing Romantic Relationships," *Communication Research* 31 (2004): 173. Tara M. Emmers-Sommer and Mike Allen, "HIV and AIDS: Toward Increased Awareness and Understanding of Prevention and Education Research Using Meta-Analysis," *Communication Studies* 52, no. 2 (2001): 127. Sarah Murnen, Perot Annette, and Donn Bryne, "Coping with Unwanted Sexual Activity: Normative Responses, Situational Determinants, and Individual Differences," *Journal of Sexual Research* 26 (1989).

26. Carolyn Clawson and Marla Reese-Weber, "The Amount and Timing of Parent-Adolescent Sexual Communication as Predictors of Late Adolescent Sexual Risk-Taking Behaviors," *Journal of Sex Research* 40 (2003): 256. T. D. Fisher, "Parent-Child Communication about Sex and Young Adolescents' Sexual Knowledge and Attitudes," *Adolescence* 21, no. 83 (1986). Mary J. Nolin and Karen K. Petersen, "Gender Differences in Parent-Child Communication about Sexuality: An Exploratory Study," *Journal of Adolescent Research* 7, no. 1 (1992). Bianca L. Guzman, Michelle Schlehofer-Sutton, and Christina M. Villanueva, "Let's Talk about Sex: How Comfortable Discussions about Sex Impact Teen Sexual Behavior," *Journal of Health Communication* 8 (2003).

27. Charles Marwick, "Survey Says Patients Expect Little Physician Help on Sex," *Journal of the American Medical Association* 281 (1999). N. Ryder, D. Ivens, and C. Sabin, "The Attitude of Patients towards Medical Students in a Sexual Health Clinic," *Sexually Transmitted Infections* 81, no. 5 (2005). Roxanne Parrott, Ashley Duggan, and Veronica Duncan, "Promoting Patients' Full and

Honest Disclosures during Conventions with Health Caregivers," in *Balancing the Secrets of Private Disclosures*, ed. Sandra Petronio (Mahwah, NJ: Lawrence Erlbaum Associates, 2000).

28. Rebecca Welch Cline, K. Freeman, and S. Johnson, "Talk among Sexual Partners about AIDS: Interpersonal Communication for Risk Reduction or Risk Enhancement?" *Health Communication* 4 (1992).

29. Eva S. Lefkowitz and Graciela Espinosa-Hernandez, "Sex-Related Communication with Mothers and Close Friends during the Transition to University," *Journal of Sex Research* 44 (2007). Christine E. Rittenour and Melanie Booth-Butterfield, "College Students' Sexual Health: Investigating the Role of Peer Communication," *Qualitative Research Reports in Communication* 7 (2006).

30. Susan Sprecher, Gardenia Harris, and Adena Meyers, "Perceptions of Sources of Sex Education and Targets of Sex Communication: Sociodemographic and Cohort Effects," *Journal of Sex Research* 45 (2008).

31. Lefkowitz and Espinosa-Hernandez, "Sex-Related Communication with Mothers."

32. Jennifer Cleary, Richard Barhman, Terry MacCormack, and Ed Herold, "Discussing Sexual Health with a Partner: A Qualitative Study with Young Women," *Canadian Journal of Human Sexuality* 11 (2002): 117–132.

33. Mike Allen, Tara Emmers-Sommer, and Tara Crowell, "Couples Negotiating Safer Sex Behaviors: A Meta-Analysis of the Impact of Conversation and Gender," in *Interpersonal Communication Research: Advances through Meta-Analysis*, ed. Raymond W. Preiss, Barbara Mae Gayle, and Nancy A. Burrell (Mahwah, NJ: Lawrence Erlbaum Associates, 2002), 266.

34. Perloff, *Persuading People*, 38.

35. Allen et al., "Couples Negotiating Safer Sex Behaviors," 263.

36. Diane diMauro, *Sexuality Research in the United States: An Assessment of the Social and Behavioral Sciences* (New York: Social Science Research Council, 1995), 3.

37. Ibid.

38. Cleary et al., "Discussing Sexual Health," 118.

39. C. Veronica Smith, "In Pursuit of 'Good' Sex: Self-Determination and the Sexual Experience," *Journal of Social and Personal Relationships* 24 (2007).

40. Michael, "Private Sex and Public Policy," 487.

41. Sprecher and McKinney, *Sexuality*.

42. Sonia L. Davison, Robin J. Bell, Maria LaChina, Samantha L. Holden, and Susan R. Davis, "Sexual Function in Well Women: Stratification by Sexual Satisfaction, Hormone Use, and Menopause Status," *Journal of Sexual Medicine* 5, no. 5 (2008).

43. Rossella E. Nappi, Kathrin Wawra, and Sonja Schmitt, "Hypoactive Sexual Desire Disorder in Postmenopausal Women," *Gynecological Endocrinology* 22, no. 6 (2006). Raymond C. Rosen and Stanley Althof, "Impact of Premature Ejaculation: The Psychological, Quality of Life, and Sexual Relationship Consequences," *Journal of Sexual Medicine* 5, no. 6 (2008).

CHAPTER 2

Our Current Sexual Climate: Sex and Society

Two college professors sat having coffee and discussing the impact of the television show and movie *Sex and the City* on society and, most especially, on their students. Dr. Green and Dr. Hill both had watched the television show and had different opinions on whether the depictions of sex and sex talk on the show were negative or positive. Dr. Hill said, "So many of our students watched the show! What really bothers me about it is the fact that many of my students were just 14 years old when they started watching *Sex and the City*. According to the definition of pornography, the show is definitely erotica, probably porn. They not only showed full frontal nudity of both men and women, they graphically discussed and, in my opinion, advocated for such topics as oral sex and anal sex, and showed graphic lesbian sex and heterosexual sex. I think it is sending the wrong message to women—promiscuity is great!"

Dr. Green responded, "I agree that the show is probably inappropriate for teenage girls, but they have to learn about these things somewhere. Don't forget about the episodes where Charlotte gets a sexually transmitted infection (STI), crabs from a summer fling, and Samantha gets tested for HIV. These were important messages for people to see. But on a much larger societal level, I think that this show was completely liberating for women and men. The female characters had open, honest, and frank discussion about sex with one another. It brought to light many topics for people to discuss. Sex is natural, it is not bad. And it showed women in charge of their own sexuality, not having sex to please men or for any other reason than pure gratification. It challenges all our notions about sexual double standards that purport men should have casual sex and enjoy sex and women should remain more pure. Come on! This is the 21st century. The material in *Sex and the City* is a reflection of society and does not directly form peoples' beliefs and opinions."

Dr. Hill replied, "I think media does a lot more than 'reflect society'—I think it creates social norms. And the norms that *Sex and the City* advocates are unhealthy for women and for men. Remember when we first started teaching? Students dated, now they just hook up. Yes, they had sex, but mostly in relationships, and women certainly did not have as many sexual partners. I just read an article about how teenagers have one of the highest rates of sexually transmitted infections of any age group in the country. Teenagers! I think *Sex and the City* and other shows like it are setting our cultural norms and girls follow them. Look at how many women loved the show—it was a huge hit. That's not for nothing. What else does *Sex and the City* teach women about sex? About men? Plus, they only openly talked about sex with one another and rarely with the people they were actually having sex with. Ultimately, it is degrading to women. The reality is that casual sex is more dangerous for women emotionally and physically. Women can get pregnant. Also, I think they are simply more emotionally vested in sexual partners than men."

"Look," an exasperated Dr. Hill says, "I am not saying every message in *Sex and the City* is great. The women are compulsive shoppers and they send a bad message about consumerism—that it is OK to go into debt to look good and you have to have expensive products to look good. And looking good is the ultimate goal for a woman. Another problematic area is family; there are no scenes with family at all! But I have to disagree with you about the sex. I am not sure, but I think they always show Samantha, the promiscuous one, using condoms. They advocate safe sex. People are going to have sex, and at least they are openly talking about it on the show. They address the good, the bad, and the ugly of sex. So many of my students told me that they started to have more conversations about sex with their friends, parents, and even boyfriends after watching a good episode. The show sent the message out, and a lot more people are going to get the message about sex from shows like this rather than in a sex education class in high school or awkward talks with their parents."

The professors hit on many current debates among media studies professors and professionals. How much do the media influence us? In what ways do the media influence us? In particular, how do the media inform our sexual relationships? If you think about it, how do we learn to talk about sex—about romance and romantic relationships, power relations, and social gender roles, and even how to have sex? How do we go about the business of making it all happen? Is there any force that influences our daily lives more than media? Undoubtedly, family, friends, work colleagues, and teachers all have a significant impact, but over time, media may have the most significant influence of all. How often to you compare real life with depictions of various aspects of life in the media? How much of your time is spent consuming media? How many of your conversations revolve around media events? It is common to hear people refer to things on TV and use them as comparisons for their own lives. Media are particularly influential when it comes to such intimate topics as sex, relationships, and sex talk because these acts are private, and we cannot model them based on our own real-life observations. While children and adolescents learn many things from their parents, generally, parents do not model appropriate sexual behaviors—they certainly cannot model something like a first sexual experience, so people turn to the media. The most frequently Googled how-to questions are "how to kiss" and "how to flirt." It is reasonable to conclude that sexually inexperienced people use TV and other forms of media as a guide to form scripts about how sexual experiences should go: how to kiss on the first date, how to handle more than one sexual partner, how to break up with someone, how to attract attention from the opposite sex, and the list could go on for a long time.[1]

Other researchers are interested in investigating the relationship between sexual attraction and the influence of celebrities. As you will read in this book, people are more sexually attracted to those who have a high status among peers; it is even called the *celebrity effect*, and it can be just as helpful as good looks or access to assets when attracting the opposite sex. What we do not know is if women who copy a specific look in the mass media attract more attention. Is a woman who copies the hairstyle, makeup, mannerisms, and clothing of a celebrity more attractive to men? On a related note, do men who see women on television find women in real life who emulate or look like them more attractive? In other words, just how much do the mass media influence what we consider to be attractive in a sexual partner?

The relationships that people sometimes develop and maintain with medial personalities or fictional characters are called *parasocial relationships*. Alan Rubin, a professor who teaches courses at Kent State University in the uses and effects of the media, believes that parasocial interaction is a normal response to media exposure, as long as people realize that they are one-sided relationships and that they do not replace real interpersonal interactions. People often experience a sense of friendship with TV characters based on feelings of similarity, attraction, and empathy for characters. Dr. Rubin explains that many media personalities intentionally use informal gestures and conversational styles that mirror interpersonal interactions to induce parasocial relationships.[2] This effect has been heightened with the influx of interactive celebrity Web sites and other forms of media such as Facebook or Twitter. By increasing their sense of personal closeness with celebrities, and therefore some of their fictional characters, people are even more vulnerable to their influences.

HYPODERMIC NEEDLE/DIRECT EFFECTS THEORY OF MEDIA VERSUS CULTIVATION THEORY

One of the underlying arguments that Dr. Hill and Dr. Green were having in the opening vignette involved the extent to which media influence people's actions and behaviors: do the media indirectly or directly influence people? People who believe in the concept of direct effects think that the mass media work like a hypodermic needle, directly injecting media messages, norms, beliefs, and behaviors into noncritical consumers. For example, researchers have been trying to establish a link between hard-core pornography and sexual violence for years but have been unable to do so; rather, they can count the number and percentage of sexually violent acts against women in a pornographic movie and contend that viewing porn changes people's attitudes involving sexual violence against women, making sexual violence more acceptable or convincing men that women "want it rough" or that women really mean yes when they say no to sex. However, researchers cannot prove that porn will cause people to go out and commit rape. It is exceedingly difficult to establish a direct effect.

The alternative concept is one of indirect effects, called *cultivation theory*. This theory essentially states that media influence people indirectly. In other words, media cultivate in us a distorted perception of reality, making life seem more like the way television portrays it, rather than how it is in real life. The media blur reality and fantasy: what life is like and what life is like in movies, romance novels, and television shows.

According to cultivation theory, reality is often distorted on TV, but people tend to believe televised portrayals of life. For example, in a 2004 study of sex life on Israeli television programming, researcher Amir Hetsroni compared how depictions of sexual activity of certain age groups on television compared to real-life data.[3] He found that sexually active teens under 18 years of age were represented in 33 percent of all television programming. However, in real life, less than 23 percent of all teens less than 18 years of age were sexually active. In contrast, in real life, 47 percent of people 65 years or older reported active sex lives, whereas less than 7 percent of all television programs depicted any kind of sexual activity among this age group. He administered a survey to almost 600 people asking them to estimate amounts of sexual activity for different age groups. Those participants who were heavy television viewers (3.5 hours of television or more per day) compared to those who were light viewers (2.5 hours or less per day) had very different estimates. Heavy viewers greatly overestimated the amount of sex that teens under 18 years of age were having and underestimated the amount of sexual activity for people over the age of 65. The people who were light viewers still overestimated the amount of sex teens were having and underestimated the amount that elders were having, but they were much closer to real-life estimates.

There have been numerous studies like the one completed by Hetsroni, and they all confirm that TV does distort people's reality, especially those who consume heavy amounts of media. People who watch large amounts of TV and consume other forms of media have a distorted view of reality. Whether you believe that TV and other forms of media directly or indirectly affect people, it is indisputable that media do affect people to various degrees, depending on their individual characteristics and levels of media consumption.

THE ROLE OF CULTURE IN FORMING OUR SEXUAL NORMS AND SEXUAL SCRIPTS

Sexual scripts theory is a useful way to make sense of how culture influences the ways people talk about sex and go about having sex. Sexual scripts define behaviors that correspond with a culture's expectations about what happens when, where, how, why, and by whom. Society helps us form the sexual scripts we use. In this chapter, there is a review of the messages about sex and sexuality that we receive from the people around us, media portrayals of sex and romance, and how people use the media to learn about sex, scripts, and even love. In several ways, popular TV shows and movies have slowly replaced traditional institutions, such as school and family, as primary sources of information about personal and sexual relationships.

In sexual scripts theory, John Gagnon and William Simon, the original theorists to come up with sexual scripts, believe that scripts function as cognitive structures that help participants define a situation, organize the interpretation of events, and guide appropriate performances in situated episodes.[4] In Gagnon and Simon's seminal work, scripts are viewed as interpretive filters and guides for behavior.[5] Basically, scripts show that humans use a set of guidelines or beliefs (i.e., a script) in directing behavior and ordering experience in the same way that an actor uses a script on the stage. The script is the actor's construction of stage reality. Communication is essential as it is necessary for the enactment of sexual scripts.[6] Communication enables participants to negotiate changes in scripts that are responsive to individual, relational, and situational features. Ongoing communication allows individuals to clarify the meaning of scripts, which results in possible changes in the interaction. People form and then internalize scripts as they try to make sense out of the world by cognitively assimilating and organizing personal experiences. This basic process is influenced by reinforcement, modeling, and rehearsal opportunities—which occur within a particular social environment. Scripting theory posits that sexuality is learned from culturally available "sexual scripts" that define what counts as sex, how to recognize sexual situations, and what to do in relational and sexual encounters.[7] The theory of scripts broadens the conceptualization of sexuality to encompass both its social dimensions and the relational contexts in which sexuality emerges (e.g., within romantic, dating, or courtship relationships). Basically, scripts take into account that sex and sex talk are influenced by culture as well as individual personalities.

Sexual scripts are not exactly the same for people who share a culture as cultural influences are only one part of how we make sense of the world. People have interpersonal differences based on religion, family, schooling, region of the country they live in, the sexual norms held by their friends, and even how individuals think about the world. According to Gagnon and Simon, we can determine behavioral outcomes on three levels of sexual scripts: cultural, interpersonal, and intrapsychic—it is our culture as well as our individual personalities that influence how we will act. Cultural scenarios are assemblies of social norms external to the individual. Cultural scenarios function as guides for sexual behavior by specifying appropriate objects, aims, and desirable qualities in relationships. Cultural scenarios are the societal norms and narratives that provide guidelines for sexual conduct, thereby broadly indicating appropriate partners and sex acts, where and when to perform those acts, and even what emotions and feelings are appropriate. These scenarios are sufficiently abstract and generalized that their specific application in particular contexts may be unclear.

Social convention and personal desire converge in interpersonal script scenarios. In interpersonal scripts, participants invoke cultural symbols to engage socially. Thus actors engaged in sexual interactions create interpersonal scripts that translate abstract cultural scenarios into scripts appropriate to particular situations. Interpersonal scripts, then, are the strategies for carrying out an individual's own sexual wishes with regard to the actual or anticipated responses of another person. Intrapsychic scripts express an individual's motivation. Intrapsychic scripts are a part of sexual arousal and concern a person's individual sexual desires and preferences.[8] "The intrapsychic script is a person's sexual fantasies, the sequence of acts, postures, objects, and gestures that elicit and sustain sexual arousal."[9] While interpersonal scripts can be seen as "sexual dialogues" with others, intrapsychic scripts are sexual dialogues with the self. Thus actors engaged in sexual interactions create interpersonal scripts that translate abstract cultural scenarios into scripts appropriate to particular situations. Interpersonal scripts, then, are the strategies for carrying out an individual's own sexual wishes with regard to the actual or anticipated responses of another person. Scripts, particularly cultural scripts, can be very helpful for people, particularly in the courtship phase of a relationship. During relationship initiation, there is a good deal of ambiguity and uncertainty. People may be worried about the impression they are making on another person, if the other person is sexually attractive (and it is reciprocated), and overall, wondering how they should act. Scripts help reduce the uncertainty and resulting anxiety by providing people appropriate roles, letting them know in a general sense how they should act. Scripts also let people know what they should expect.

Scripts can have a deep effect on people and their actions. For example, part of why there is so much unprotected sex in the United States is based on the script about sexual spontaneity. The current pattern of sexual interaction scripts is often predicated on a lack of planning and foresight because sexual encounters are not viewed as something a person should plan. We are instilled with a need to feel spontaneity, and many times, an individual may feel a desire not to have a conversational plan or script developed because such a plan means confronting one's sexual desires and behaviors. We like to believe or pretend that sex happens spontaneously because it's more natural and perhaps more intense because it "just happens," something frequently reinforced by sexual relationships on TV or in the movies. TV sitcoms and movies often make fun of couples that plan sex in advance—"Let's have sex on Saturday"—or discuss their "weekly sex appointment." These couples are portrayed as pathetic, not very sexy, and certainly not to be envied. However, the reality for most couples, particularly those with young children, is that they must make plans to have sex because spontaneous sex is unrealistic. For these couples, if they do not make time to have sex, they probably will not have it.

THE FIRST DATE SCRIPT

Let us look at a popular script that we should all understand: the first date script. What should a first date be like? We all have some idea about this, mostly based on media portrayals of the first date. Even with the recent advent of "hooking up," one could argue that dating has been the primary manner in which courtship in the United States has taken place since the 1920s, and even people who have never dated share a vision of what a first date ought to be like. First dates are of particular importance: for one, they may be a relationship turning point, when people decide to move from a platonic relationship to a romantic one. Because the first date is literally a test to see if people are going to move to a romantic relationship, there is a high level of ambiguity—the unknown. For these reasons, we often remember first dates and place special importance on them. Although it may seem like we live in a diverse and ever changing society and that there is no universally shared first date script, research has shown that at least college students do have a common understanding of how a first date should go. First date behaviors that are common and expected include grooming for the date, engaging in small talk, and adhering to gender roles.

According to professors Mary Claire Morr and Paul Mongeau, who wrote an article titled "First-Date Expectations: The Impact of Sex of Initiator, Alcohol Consumption, and Relationship Type,"[10] "first date scripts consistently depict men as taking an active role and women as taking a passive one. The man is expected to initiate the date, plan the date activities, drive, pay for the date, and initiate sexual intimacy, whereas women are expected to wait for the man to initiate sexual contact and then decide whether or not to accept/reject a date's sexual advances."[11] Behaviors in the first date script are consistent with traditional sexual scripts in which men are expected to be the sexual initiators and women the sexual gatekeepers.[12] First date scripts with a male initiator and a female recipient are so ingrained in the United States that even when ordered to have role reversal in an experiment, many people could not do it.[13]

So imagine your first date script—most people's are surprising similar. Man invites the woman to dinner and a movie. He picks her up, drives them to their destinations, pays for dinner and the movie (the woman should offer to pay, but then he politely insists on picking up the check), then drives her home, and perhaps they will kiss if the date went well. This is a fairly standard first date scenario. If we really look at it, it becomes clear how culture has influenced our idea of a first date, as variations of this very scenario are reenacted again and again in our popular culture images.

Recently, there has been an influx of reality-based shows about first dates and finding mates showing more exciting first date scenarios than dinner and a movie. In part, this is due to the fact that a television camera cannot follow a couple into a movie theater. That would be one boring show! So the televised dates usually show some off-beat date such as karate lessons or a cooking class or rollerblading, and then a meal. It will be interesting to see how these shows influence people's first date expectations. Last, because we have some relatively new venues for dating, such as the Internet sites e-Harmony or Match.com, individual conceptions of first dates may be changing. You see many "TV couples" that meet on the Internet establishing rules. One rule may be that they just meet for coffee so they are not stuck with the person for a whole meal if they do not hit it off with that person. Norms about Internet dating in movies and on TV started as far back as 1998 with the Tom Hanks and Meg Ryan hit movie *You've Got Mail.*

LEVEL OF SEXUAL CONTENT ON TV

How much sexual content is in the media? What kind of sexual content is in the media? Researchers who study mediated sexual messages literally count the number of sexual messages/images and the kinds of sexual messages and images shown in all kinds of mass media formats, including movies, television shows, magazines, musical lyrics, music videos, video games, and on numerous different Internet sites. Within these contexts, researchers have broken down the categories into specific genres (rap music) or time slots (primetime television vs. daytime television) and different kinds of programming (soap operas, dramas, and sitcoms). Other researchers have examined sexual content across the entire television environment.[14] Results from all different kinds of studies confirm that the amount of sexual content in the mass media is considerable and has been increasing exponentially over the years.

A Kaiser Family Foundation report offers the most comprehensive and recent analysis of sexual content in the media. The study leader, Dr. Dale Kunkel, and his team performed detailed analyses in 1999 and then repeated the analysis in 2005.[15] Kunkel defined sexual content as "any depiction of sexual activity, sexually suggestive behavior, or talk about sexuality or sexual activity,"[16] which accounts for different types of sexual dialogue and a wide variety of sexual behaviors, ranging from kissing and physical flirting to depictions of sexual intercourse. Kunkel's group and others have confirmed that the verbal and visual references to sexual activity were numerous, especially in programming viewed by adolescents, and that rates of sexual content have increased dramatically over time.

The Kaiser Family Foundation report showed that the percentage of television programs containing sexual content significantly rose from 56 percent in the 1997–98 television seasons to 70 percent of shows in 2004–5. In the 2004–5 TV season, approximately 1 in 10 programs portrayed sexual intercourse. However, these depictions are rarely explicit; rather, the most frequent sexual behaviors take the form of passionate kissing or touching of others' intimate body parts. In most cases, intercourse is strongly implied, rather than directly shown. However, when intercourse and other explicit sexual behaviors are shown on television, people really pay attention, particularly adolescents. The authors explained in the report why young people pay particular attention to explicit depictions of sex:

> Because of this unique status of intercourse among all sexual behaviors, its context of presentation may be distinct from the overall pattern of messages about sexuality in the media. Moreover, as compared with such behaviors as kissing and petting, intercourse carries with it higher risks of spreading sexually transmitted infections and pregnancy. The intimate nature of this behavior can also carry heightened emotional and social implications. The fact that adolescents are likely to pay especially close attention to portrayals of intercourse makes the examination of messages about this behavior important.[17]

The context of sexual behavior in the media has also been assessed in terms of whether sex is portrayed as a recreational or relational activity,[18] whether sexual partners are married,[19] and how frequently references to sexual risk or responsibility (e.g., contraception, pregnancy, STIs) are made.[20] There is more talk about sex on TV than depictions of people having sex. Studies have consistently shown that talk about sex and sexuality is more common than sexual behaviors, with more than two-thirds of television shows containing sexual talk.[21] Studies also have found that sexual behavior typically takes place between unmarried adults.[22] Indeed, according to a 2009 comprehensive content analysis study by media experts Keren Eyal and Keli Finnerty,[23] most of the people having sex on TV are not married—only 15 percent of the depictions of sexual intercourse took place between married couples. Of the remaining couples,

29 percent were in an established unmarried sexual relationship with one another, 32 percent did not have a previously established sexual relationship, and 14 percent of couples had just met. Kunkel found that although more than half of the couples who engage in sexual intercourse on television are in an established relationship, 1 in 10 are couples who have met only recently, and one-quarter of TV couples do not start or maintain a relationship after having sex.[24]

Furthermore, analyses showed that sex between characters who share different relational statuses (i.e., married, established, not established, and those who have just met) do not differ in the extent to which they portray any kind of consequence. This is surprising given that sex with a stranger places individuals at greater risk of experiencing negative emotional outcomes, such as guilt or regret,[25] and negative physical outcomes, such as unplanned pregnancy or STI contraction.[26]

The fact that most sex on TV has no negative consequences is important and related to a concept developed in the 1920s and 1930s by Floyd Allport called *pluralistic ignorance*. This is when a person believes that his private attitudes, beliefs, or judgments differ from the norm exhibited by the public behavior of others.[27] Each individual who believes that she is different from the group wishes to be a part of the group and therefore publicly conforms to the norm, believing that she is the only one in the group that is conflicted over her private beliefs and public behavior. Later in the 1950s, Katz and Lazarsfeld further developed the concept by conducting research and found that group members believed that the opinion leaders and the most popular people in their group actually approved of the behavior, while the individual is really going along with the behavior because of a desire to fit in, even though he may feel uncomfortable with the behavior and feel bad about it privately. Numerous studies have shown that people consistently overestimate the amount of sex they believe their peers are having, particularly among adolescents and young adults and those involved in casual sex. When the media create false norms about sexual practices involving frequency of sex, duration of sex, and even safety, they can impact the actual behaviors of people in countless ways, even if the people are uncomfortable with the behaviors.

Pluralistic ignorance is common for men and women when it comes to dating beliefs and the timing of sex. Both men and women thought that the normal, average, representative person of their same sex had more open-minded ideas and expectations about sex than they did.[28] Both sexes believed that the average person would have sex or expect sex sooner in a relationship than they would. What about the importance of attraction to the opposite sex? Men and women believed that the average man and woman would expect intercourse with someone with whom they were emotionally involved but to whom they felt no attraction, even though 50 percent of those surveyed personally stated that they would not expect or want sex in this kind of situation. An even smaller number reported actually having sex in this situation. In situations where there was no physical or emotional connection, very few people reported that they would personally expect sex, but they thought that the average man or woman would expect sex. It is clear that most men and women greatly overestimate the amount of sex expected in different situations. Where do people get such ideas? Of course, we think of the media right away. Although, as discussed in this chapter, it cannot be proven that the media cause these kinds of beliefs, it certainly seems like common sense that the media would be at least part of the influence.

DEPICTIONS OF MASCULINITY AND FEMININITY IN THE MEDIA

Television provides viewers with detailed information guiding how girls/women and boys/men should think, feel, and behave in romantic and sexual relationships. Child development and social psychology experts Kay Bussey and Albert Bandura believe that the media play a major role in modeling of gender roles, as television, video games, and books portray men "as directive, venturesome, enterprising, and pursuing engaging occupations and recreational activities. In contrast, women are usually shown as acting in dependent, unambitious, and emotional ways."[29] Central to the idea of modeling gender roles is Bandura's idea of *vicarious observation*. The "televised vicarious influence has dethroned the primacy of direct experience. Whether it be thought patterns, values, attitudes, or styles of behavior, life increasingly models the media."[30] Cultural and mediated images of masculinity, femininity, and sexuality undoubtedly perpetuate dominant ideologies, but the stable, recurrent patterns of televised images may play a particularly significant role in fostering gender roles. Therefore, according to Bandura's theory, the fictional televised sexual experiences of characters on TV replace real experiences of people. Because of this, and the fact that media messages are continuous and show relatively uniform depictions of sexual experiences and conversations, we can say that not only does TV influence how people talk about sex, but it does so in unrealistic ways.

Portrayals of male sexuality in the media are pervasive, and the messages are clear and unilateral: accumulating sexual experience with women is an important, desirable, and even a necessary component of masculinity, and boys/men should attain sexual experience by any means possible. Indeed, Kunkel found that in several TV programs, male characters used forceful or deceitful strategies to persuade female characters to engage in sexual activity or to catch glimpses of them unclothed. In contrast, feminine courtship strategies encouraged girls/women to seduce boys/men by exploiting their bodies and dressing in tight, revealing clothing, even though, on the same TV shows, these behaviors were devalued and seen as a sign of female characters' sexual indiscretion or impropriety. Such depictions reveal the challenge that girls face when they are encouraged both to conform to omnipresent conventions of femininity and sexual purity and perform active gatekeeping on boys' "uncontrollable" sexual desire.[31] Television offers mutually impoverished constructs of male and female sexuality, which may ultimately preclude boys' ability to say no to sex and girls' ability to say yes. From television, then, viewers learn that boys/men and girls/women need to be in a state of constant vigilance and must regulate their sexuality. Whereas boys must constantly work to construct and assert their masculinity, girls walk the precarious line between making themselves sexually available to men and being appropriately demure—the tension at the heart of femininity. We also learn that when it comes to communicating about sex, people on TV do not talk about sex in meaningful ways; most of the talk around sex is supposed to be humorous. There are countless sexual innuendos and jokes on TV. It is interesting that the situation comedies with the most vulgar sexual jokes tend to be the most popular. For example, the CBS situation comedy that features one vulgar sexual joke after another, *Two and a Half Men*, has maintained a top 10 spot on the Nielsen rating for years, one of the only half-hour TV sitcoms to do so.

According to author Lynn Phillips, there are additional traditional cultural gender scripts for women depicted in the media, including the "Pleasing Woman," the "Cosmo Chick," and the "Together Woman." The "Pleasing Woman" is selfless and sacrifices her own desires for the benefit of others.[32] In addition, she is sexually innocent, delicate, and moral; however, her appearance and behaviors are sexually pleasing to men. The pleasing women deny their own sexual desires, yet are encouraged to be the object of desire for men. It is up to the woman to safeguard her sexual purity from men in this case. The "Together Woman" has it all, is self-autonomous, and seeks pleasure equal to that of men's in her sexual encounters. She is often depicted in TV shows such as *Sex and the City*, taking sex when she wants it and handling all the emotional and physical fallout with ease. The "Cosmo Chick" is named for *Cosmopolitan* magazine, whose issues are filled with images of women who are autonomous, sexually experienced (and good at it), sophisticated, and encouraged to participate in sex outside of relationships. At the same time, the "Cosmo Chick" is encouraged to find the line between the positive behaviors and negative behaviors that would have them appear to be slutty, cheap, sufferers of low self-esteem, or needy when it comes to men. Personal responsibility regarding sex is not part of the "Cosmo Chick" script. One could say that women are encouraged to act like men to gain male attention.

SEX TALK IN THE MEDIA

How do media affect how we talk about sex? One could argue that sex is everywhere in the mainstream media: on TV, in movies, and in advertisements and magazines. I believe this is true, but the problem is that very few of these media outlets offer meaningful information about sex talk. It is ironic in that as a culture, we have trivialized sex, while at the same time, we have endowed it with too much importance. Indeed, we trivialize it and use sex to provide humor and jokes in countless media formats. As demonstrated in the analysis of the sexual content on TV, overwhelmingly, media fail to provide positive or educational images of sex and rarely show images of essential and basic safe-sex behaviors like abstinence, discussions of previous partners, getting tested, and/or using condoms.

The British government was interested in finding out if and to what extent the media affect youth and their attitudes about sex to make important policy decisions. They commissioned media experts Sarah Bragg and David Buckingham to study the phenomenon. Bragg and Buckingham presented their findings to British government in a comprehensive report and also published the data in a book titled *Young People, Sex and the Media*. One of the most important things that Bragg and Buckingham found is that people, particularly young people, are learning more and more about how to talk about sex with friends, family, and sexual partners from popular television dramas.[33] Why? Young people explained that they *prefer* TV for sex education (particularly soap operas) over educational messages by parents or teachers because they believe that these media narratives are often more informative, less embarrassing, and more attuned to their needs and concerns.[34]

Also, while the intended messages about sex may be clear to most adults, youths had a hard time identifying messages about sex and relationships in the media, and when they did identify messages, they were not uniform or clear. For example, the story line shows a negative consequence to sexual activity, such as a girl has sex with a boy, then he breaks up with her and spreads rumors about her, and she gets a bad reputation and becomes depressed. To adults, the message would be quite clear and clearly negative, yet youths had a hard time identifying the message, and if they could identify a message, it was rarely the same message other youths identified. Bragg and Buckingham concluded that media messages about sex were mixed and required that people make up their own minds about the intent of the messages. Adults have reason to be optimistic because Bragg and Buckingham also found that young people were actually fairly savvy media consumers and became more critical consumers of media as they consumed more media and became older. Indeed, they found that with sexual messages, most of the young people focused on the messages that highlighted the importance of trust, fidelity, and mutual respect in sexual encounters.

Another theme about sex talk in media is that men should start conversations about sex and, while women should be more passive about sex talk, they should also be experts on relationship issues. The traditional sexual script dictates that women are "not supposed to indicate directly their sexual interest or engage freely in sexuality" and that men are "supposed to take the initiative even when a woman indicates verbally that she is unwilling to have sex (presumably because of the male belief that a woman's initial resistance is only token)."[35] This script involves the idea of *token resistance*, which has been around in popular culture for a long time. Depictions of token resistance are found in Louisa May Alcott's *Little Women* and Jane Austen's *Pride and Prejudice*. Many popular television programs, and especially pornography, incorporate this theme into their portrayals of sexually active couples. Women are not supposed to want sex, let alone talk about it. So the idea that women are the nurturers and responsible for communication in relationships is at direct odds with the idea of token resistance and the lack of expression of female desire. Therefore it is very difficult for women to talk about sex and express their sexuality. They are supposed to wait for the man to take the lead. Male sexual scripts discourage men from talking about feelings and sexuality. The result is limited meaningful communication about sex between people. Interestingly, research about token resistance shows that men are more likely to report token resistance than women, which is completely contrary to the stereotype depicted on TV and in the movies.[36] In other words, men reported that they were likely to say no when they really wanted to have sex and had every intention of engaging in sexual activity. On the whole, women reported saying no because they felt like it was the right thing to do, to be a "good girl," even if their bodies wanted to have sex—and they did not engage in sexual activities. In real life, when women say no, they mean it.

SAFE SEX AND SEXUAL CONSEQUENCES ON TV

There are many emotional and physical consequences to sex, yet these consequences are rarely depicted on TV and even less frequently in the movies. Keren Eyal and Keli Finnerty, two communication researchers, have long been gathering data on the amount and nature of sexual content in the media—in particular, the depiction of consequences that occur when TV characters engage in sexual intercourse. Eyal and Finnerty used the definition of *consequences* provided by the Kaiser Family Foundation study. Consequences included (1) the mention or depiction of sexual precautions (e.g., the use of birth control methods); (2) the mention or depiction of risks and/or negative consequences of sexual intercourse (e.g., HIV/AIDS or other STI contraction or the mention of an unplanned or unwanted pregnancy); and (3) the mention or depiction of sexual patience, the importance of waiting to have sex, or maintaining one's virginity. Eyal and Finnerty contend that "the portrayal of such consequences of intercourse on television can affect viewers' attitudes toward sexual intercourse; their outcome and risk expectancies; and, in turn, their sexual behavior."[37] In their latest study, published in 2009, Eyal and Finnerty analyzed 152 TV shows and found that almost half of all shows (45%) included one act of sexual intercourse, and one in five shows (20%) included more than two intercourse acts. On the whole, most programs with sexual intercourse portrayals averaged two intercourse acts per program. Use of sexual precautions is mentioned or depicted in approximately 4 percent of acts, and risks or negative consequences of sexuality and concerns with sexual patience are each included in only 0.4 percent of acts.

In the 1970s, NBC was the first of the major networks to depict rather than imply sex on television. Incredulously, NBC prohibited the use of birth control for its characters because "birth control, after all, meant characters had planned sexual encounters, rather than just being swept up in passionate moments."[38] So NBC executives decided that it was acceptable to show unplanned and unsafe sex. We can see what this means for communication about sex, and safe sex, in particular. Major networks, while depicting explicit sex scenes, banned advertisements for condoms— many of them still ban condom advertisements. In 2009, Fox and CBS banned a Trojan condom advertisement because it highlighted contraception messages rather than health messages. Yet, on these same networks, you can see advertisements for Viagra and Valtrex (a medication for genital herpes). The televised message about sex is clear: it is OK to have sex, as long as it is unsafe and unplanned.

Eyal and Finnerty also found that TV characters often cheat and feel no remorse or suffer any consequences. In fact, 25 percent of all sexual acts on TV involved cheating. The vast majority (92%) of acts were consensual or mutually agreed upon by both participants. The loss of virginity was also in 5 percent of sex acts for at least one TV character. Of the characters whose age could be discerned (90% of all characters), four out of five (83%) were adults older than 25 years of age. One of every 10 characters (11%) was a young adult, and 5 percent were teenagers. Of the 606 identifiable consequences that were shown, most (73%) resulted in positive emotional outcomes of happiness and excitement. In contrast, only 27 percent were found to result in negative emotions such as guilt or regret. Pregnancy was depicted in only 7 percent of all consequences, and even then, approximately one-half of the characters were happy about the pregnancy. Not surprisingly, not one show depicted characters getting STIs or HIV/AIDS from unsafe sex.

In 2004, Jennifer Stevens Aubrey analyzed the content of prime-time programs that feature teens and found that more than 33 percent of the sex scenes had some kind of consequence for teens who engaged in sexual activities (including talk).[39] Approximately 88 percent of the consequences were negative and did not focus on physical health issues; rather, the negative consequences were emotional (disappointment, guilt, anxiety) and social (humiliation, rejection, ostracism for girls). Less than 20 percent of the consequences included a mention of pregnancy or STIs, and less than 10 percent involved any kind of punishment from others for having sex. These findings are even more profound in movies. A 2005 study by media scholar Amy Chu looked at the consequences of sex in the most popular movies in the last 20 years and found that almost 90 percent of all movies showed that sexual intercourse had no consequences (no pregnancy, no STIs, no emotional or social ramifications).[40] In fact, Chu could not find one popular movie that showed an STI transmission or unplanned pregnancy.

As discussed in this chapter, safe-sex practices are rarely shown on many television shows and movies. Additionally, the dominant pattern of sexual interaction is often predicated on a lack of planning and foresight because sexual encounters are not viewed as something a person should plan. Indeed, with sex on the screen, there is a palpable, almost forced spontaneity. Often fictional couples do not even make it to the bedroom. This makes viewers feel like it is more natural and desirable for sex to be spontaneous and out of control (and comfortable on a staircase). This is the message we get from mainstream media as well as pornography. Great sex should be unplanned, spur of the moment, and without conversation. Sex on TV and in movies is often depicted as wonderful and always highly satisfying—partners are overcome with desire, leading to sweaty, long-lasting, pleasurable sex. Unless it is a comedy about young males attempting to lose their virginity, sex is most often portrayed in an extremely positive light. The inexperienced male is mocked—many comedies, such as *The 40 Year Old Virgin*, revolve around ridiculing the sexually inept male characters.

We rarely see people on TV and in movies talking in meaningful ways about sex, let alone safe sex, unless they are joking about it. Not only do we lack role models who talk openly about safe sex, but it goes deeper, influencing our patterns of behavior with our sexual partners. Since we rarely see media characters engaging in meaningful communication about sex and safe sex, we do not feel that these are natural and comfortable conversations. Mike Allen, a communication scholar who plans safe-sex interventions, believes that "the first step in any educational intervention is literally convincing a person that having conversations does not involve the development of some type of anti-social or undesirable practice."[41]

IMPLICATIONS FOR SEX TALK: IMPROVING YOUR SEXUAL COMMUNICATION

Researchers have been studying portrayals of sexuality on TV for decades and have found a steady increase of sexual content over the years. In this chapter, I provided evidence that sexual content saturates television programs. The public opinion poll by the Kaiser Family Foundation found that over 60 percent of parents are "very concerned" about the amount of sexual content their children see. One TV commentator suggested that there is so much sex in the media now that it is no longer edgy; rather, it is almost "redundant and old fashioned" to show sex on TV, and as a society, we do not associate illicit values with sexual behavior anymore.[42] Again, it is very difficult to prove that media directly influence sexual beliefs and behaviors. What we do know is that because there is such widespread sexual content in the media (TV, movies, Internet, magazines, and music), it serves to keep sexual issues on the public agenda and on our private agendas. Media scholars like to say that "the media do not tell us what to think, but what to think about." We also know that there are relatively consistent messages across media formats about sexuality—including relationship norms and sex norms. This influences individuals' cultural, interpersonal, and intrapersonal scripts regarding communication about sex and sexual interactions. We can see how this plays out when we remember the example of our first date script. Media significantly influence how we think a sexual interaction should go.

There was also a review of numerous studies that showed that the mass media indoctrinate men and women into gender-appropriate sexual roles. Magazines, television programs, and movies frequently depict females as sexually submissive to male sexual power and dominance. Magazines targeted to young women promote passivity as a way to sexually satisfy men, and advertisements in both men's and women's magazines portray women as submissive to and dependent on men. Female sexual submission and male sexual power are also prominent themes in romance novels and mainstream literature.

One way to counter the effects of media is to become media literate. *Media literacy* is the concept that people should be able to evaluate media content critically and be able to construct accurate comparisons between media content and social reality. The idea is that if people had a more accurate and complete picture of media content, then people could better understand its effects on audience members. While most people, even young people, on some level are already critical of media messages, thinking about the media in more critical terms, especially when it comes to evaluating sexual norms and behaviors, and how this translates into communication about sex can be especially important to improve quality communication in real life.

It is also important to recognize realistic sexual norms. By understanding that the media portray unrealistic sexual expectations for men and women, people can feel better about their sex lives. People do not have terrific sex every day. By understanding and settling realistic sexual expectations between partners, you can greatly improve your sexual relationship. By using media sources such as a television program or a movie to start a discussion or continue a discussion about sex, sex talk, and expectations, sexual communication may help break the silence in a relationship. Last, it is important to recognize what is missing from television and movie messages about sex: safe-sex messages and condom use, which could prevent a host of negative consequences such as unintended pregnancies and STIs. In general, the media also lack characters that model meaningful communication about sex between partners, parents and children, and friends. Often sexual content on TV is reduced to jokes and puns, which are not necessarily bad, but if research shows that the majority of children prefer TV for sexual education, then we have to note that essential elements of a safe and meaningful sexual relationship are missing. Knowledge is power. Whether you believe Dr. Hill or Dr. Green from the opening vignette, whether you believe media have direct or indirect effects, whether you believe that the influx of sex on TV has positive or negative messages, being informed about the different views on the influence of media on sex talk is extremely important.

NOTES

1. Jane D. Brown, "Mass Media Influences on Sexuality," *Journal of Sex Research* 39 (2002).

2. Alan M. Rubin, Elizabeth M. Perse, and Robert A. Powell, "Loneliness, Parasocial Interaction and Local Television Viewing," *Human Communication Research* 12 (1985).

3. Amir Hetsroni, "Overrepresented Topics, Underrepresented Topics, and the Cultivation Effect," *Communication Research Reports* 25 (2008).

4. John Gagnon and William Simon, *Sexual Conduct: The Social Sources of Human Sexuality* (Chicago: Aldine-Atherton Press, 1973). Sandra Metts and Brian Spitzberg, "Sexual Communication in Interpersonal Contexts: A Script-Based Approach," in *Communication Yearbook*, ed. Brant Burleson (Mahwah, NJ: Lawrence Erlbaum Associates, 1996). G. P. Ginsburg, "Rules, Scripts, and Prototypes in Personal Relationships," in *Handbook of Personal Relationships*, ed. Steven Duck (London: John Wiley, 1988).

5. Gagnon and Simon, *Sexual Conduct*.

6. Metts and Spitzberg, "Sexual Communication in Interpersonal Contexts."

7. Gagnon and Simon, *Sexual Conduct*. William Simon and John Gagnon, "A Sexual Scripts Approach," in *Theories of Human Sexuality*, ed. J. H. Geer and W. O'Donahue (New York: Plenum, 1987).

8. Metts and Spitzberg, "Sexual Communication in Interpersonal Contexts."

9. Simon and Gagnon, "A Sexual Scripts Approach," 198.

10. Paul Mongeau and Mary Clair Morr, "First Date Expectations: The Impact of Sex of Initiator, Alcohol Consumption, and Relationship Type," *Communication Research* 31 (2004): 3.

11. Suzanna Rose and Irene H. Frieze, "Young Singles' Contemporary Dating Scripts," *Sex Roles* 28, no. 9 (1993): 504.

12. Marcia N. LaPlante, Naomi McCormick, and Gary G. Brannigan, "Living the Sexual Script: College Students' Views of Influence in Sexual Encounters," *Journal of Sex Research* 16, no. 4 (1980). Sandra Metts and William R. Cupach, "The Role of Communication in Human Sexuality," in *Human Sexuality: The Societal and Interpersonal Context*, ed. Kathleen McKinney and Susan

Sprecher (Westport, CT: Ablex, 1989). Metts and Spitzberg, "Sexual Communication in Interpersonal Contexts."

13. In an experiment where female college students were instructed to initiate a first date, the male recipient in the dyad ended up asking the woman out 31% of the time. For a full review of the study, see Sandra Metts and Sylvia Mikucki, "The Emotional Landscape of Romantic Relationship Initiation," in *Handbook of Relationship Initiation*, ed. Susan Sprecher, Amy Wenzel, and John Harvey (New York: Psychology Press, 2008), 238.

14. Dale Kunkel, Kirstie Cope, Wendy Jo Farinola, Emma Rollin, and Edward Donnerstein, "Sex on TV: A Biennial Report to the Kaiser Family Foundation" (Menlo Park, CA: Kaiser Family Foundation, 1999). Dale Kunkel, Kirstie Cope-Farrar, Erica Biely, Wendy Jo Farinola, and Edward Donnerstein, "Sex on TV, 2: A Biennial Report to the Kaiser Family Foundation" (Menlo Park, CA: Kaiser Family Foundation, 2001). Dale Kunkel, Keren Eyal, Keli Finnerty, Erica Biely, and Edward Donnerstein, "Sex on TV, 4" (Menlo Park, CA: Kaiser Family Foundation, 2005), 67. Deborah A. Fisher, Douglas L. Hill, Joel W. Grube, and Enid L. Gruber, "Sex on American Television: An Analysis across Program Genres and Network Types," *Journal of Broadcasting and Electronic Media* 48 (2004).

15. Kunkel et al., "Sex on TV, 4," 14. Kunkel et al., "Sex on TV." Kunkel et al., "Sex on TV, 2."

16. Kunkel et al., "Sex on TV, 4," 15. Erica Biely and Edward Donnerstein.

17. Ibid., 144. Erica Biely and Edward Donnerstein.

18. L. Monique Ward, "Talking about Sex: Common Themes about Sexuality in the Prime-Time Television Programs Children and Adolescents View Most," *Journal of Youth and Adolescence* 24, no. 5 (1995).

19. Dennis T. Lowry and Jon A. Shidler, "Prime Time TV Portrayals of Sex, 'Safe Sex' and AIDS: A Longitudinal Analysis," *Journalism Quarterly* 70, no. 3 (1993).

20. Ibid.

21. Carol J. Pardun, Kelly Ladin L'Engle, and Jane D. Brown, "Linking Exposure to Outcomes: Early Adolescents' Consumption of Sexual Content in Six Media," *Mass Communication and Society* 8 (2005). Kunkel et al., "Sex on TV, 4," 167. Erica Biely and Edward Donnerstein. Fisher et al., "Sex on American Television."

22. Bradley Greenberg and Rick Busselle, *Soap Operas and Sexual Activity* (Menlo Park, CA: Kaiser Family Foundation, 1994). Bradley Greenberg, C. Stanley, M. Siemicki, C. Heeter, A. Soderman, and R. Linsangan, "Sex Content on Soaps and Prime-Time Television Series Most Viewed by Adolescents," in *Media, Sex, and the Adolescent*, ed. Bradely Greenberg, Jane Brown, and Nancy Buerkel-Rothfuss (Cresskill, NJ: Hampton, 1993).

23. Keren Eyal and Keli Finnerty, "The Portrayal of Sexual Intercourse on Television: How, Who, and with What Consequence?" *Mass Communication and Society* 12 (2009).

24. Pardun et al., "Linking Exposure to Outcomes."

25. Antonia Abbey, Lisa Thompson Ross, Donna McDuffie, and Pam McAuslan, "Alcohol and Dating Risk Factors for Sexual Assault among College Women," *Psychology of Women Quarterly* 20, no. 1 (1996). Elizabeth L. Paul, Brian McManus, and Allison Hayes, "'Hookups': Characteristics and Correlates of College Students' Spontaneous and Anonymous Sexual Experiences," *Journal of Sex Research* 37 (2000).

26. J. A. Catania, T. J. Coates, R. Stall, H. Turner, J. Peterson, N. Hearst, M. M. Dolcini, et al., "Prevalence of AIDS-Related Risk Factors and Condom Use in the United States," *Science* 258, no. 5085 (1992).

27. T. A. Lambert, A. S. Kahn, and K. J. Apple, "Pluralistic Ignorance and Hooking Up," *Journal of Sex Research* 40, no. 2 (2003): 129.

28. L. L. Cohen and R. L. Shotland, "Timing of First Sexual Intercourse in a Relationship: Expectations, Experiences, and Perceptions of Others," *Journal of Sex Research* 33, no. 4 (1996). Study as reviewed by Lambert et al., "Pluralistic Ignorance and Hooking Up," 130.

29. Kay Bussey and Albert Bandura, "Social Cognitive Theory of Gender Development and Differentiation," *Psychological Review* 106, no. 4 (1999): 701.

30. Albert Bandura, *Social Foundations of Thought and Action: A Social Cognitive Theory* (Englewood Cliffs, NJ: Prentice Hall, 1986), 20.

31. Sandra Lee Bartky, *Femininity and Domination* (New York: Routledge, 1990).

32. Lynn M. Phillips, *Flirting with Danger: Young Women's Reflections on Sexuality and Domination* (New York: New York University Press, 2000).

33. Nancy Signorielli, "Sex on Prime-Time in the 90's," *Communication Research Reports* 17, no. 1 (2000). Nancy Signorielli, "Adolescents and Ambivalence toward Marriage: A Cultivation Analysis," *Youth and Society* 23, no. 1 (1991). C. Segrin and Robin Nabi, "Does Television Viewing Cultivate Unrealistic Expectations about Marriage?" *European Journal of Communication* 52 (2002).

34. Sarah Bragg and David Buckingham, *Young People, Sex and the Media* (Hampshire, UK: Palgrave Macmillan, 2004).

35. James V. Check and Neil M. Malamuth, "Sex Role Stereotyping and Reactions to Depictions of Stranger versus Acquaintance Rape," *Journal of Personality and Social Psychology* 45, no. 2 (1983): 344.

36. Charlene Muehlenhard and Carie Rodgers, "Token Resistance to Sex: New Perspectives on an Old Stereotype," in *Speaking of Sexuality*, ed. Kenneth Davidson and Nelwyn Moore (Los Angeles, CA: Roxbury, 2005).

37. Eyal and Finnerty, "Portrayal of Sexual Intercourse on Television," 146.

38. Elana Levine, *Wallowing in Sex: The New Sexual Culture of 1970s American Television* (Durham, NC: Duke University Press, 2007), 320.

39. Jennifer Stevens Aubrey, "Sex and Punishment: An Examination of Sexual Consequences and the Sexual Double Standard in Teen Programming," *Sex Roles* 50, no. 7 (2004).

40. Amy Chu, "Teen Movies as Sex Education Material? A Content Analysis of Popular Teen Movies in Four Decades," paper presented at the annual meeting of the International Communication Association, 2007.

41. Mike Allen, Tara M. Emmers-Sommer, and Tara L. Crowell, "Couples Negotiating Safer Sex Behaviors: A Meta-Analysis of the Impact of Conversation and Gender," in *Interpersonal Communication Research: Advances through Meta-Analysis*, ed. Raymond W. Preiss, Barbara Mae Gayle, and Nancy A. Burrell (Mahwah, NJ: Lawrence Erlbaum Associates, 2002), 267.

42. P. J. Bednarski, "Oh, Is TV Naughty," *Broadcasting and Cable* 133, no. 39 (2003): 37.

CHAPTER 3

Gender and Cultural Issues That Influence Communication about Sex

Sue and her partner Amir have been together for six years. Sue is in love with Amir, and they have lived together for four years. She talks to her best friend, Krissy, regularly on the phone. Krissy and Sue often talk about their friendship and why they like each other so much. Just the other day, Sue said, "Krissy, I just love you. You are a great friend. When I am feeling down, I know that talking to you makes me feel better. We have to see each other more, though. I love talking on the phone, especially because I can get things done at home while we are talking on the phone, but I really miss the face-to-face time." Krissy responds by saying, "Yes, I miss the face-to-face time, as well. I understand how you feel, but with my new job and the twins at home, it is just tough. Hey, remember the time we met for lunch at Julios and . . . ?" Krissy goes on to finish the story. Men are sometimes confounded by the fact that women can talk on the phone for such long periods of time and about "nothing in particular."

Sue and Krissy are comfortable talking about their relationship and do not necessarily problem solve (they don't see each other face-to-face often enough and do not make a plan to fix it) but just feel better by talking about it. However, if women try to communicate with their boyfriends or husbands about the relationship, it often doesn't go so well. Can we talk about our relationship? This statement is frequently dreaded by men and women alike because it often ends in misunderstandings or hurt feelings. Men sometimes dread the relationship conversation because they often do not see a point in talking about a relationship unless there is a problem to solve, whereas many women often derive pleasure in simply talking about their relationships. A miscommunication may occur between men, who do not think there is a problem with the relationship and therefore do not want to talk about the relationship, and women, who just wanted to talk and may jump to the conclusion that there really is a problem in the relationship because their partners do not want to talk about it. Before this miscommunication, the woman did not think there was a problem with the relationship. This is an excellent example of how men and women communicate differently.

I wrote my dissertation on the experiences of Indian immigrant women and published subsequent articles on their views of acculturation and sexuality. One of my closest friends inspired me to explore this topic. She grew up in India and had an arranged marriage. She had met her husband three times (all supervised) before she married him and moved to the United States. How people come together and get married greatly varies within cultures, and it is an interesting phenomenon to study. I often ask my students, how many of you would trust your parents to pick out a suitable spouse? I ask friends my age, how many of you would probably have been better off had you let your parents pick a spouse for you? I always have a few students who do say, "Yes, I would trust my parents to arrange a marriage for me; heck, it would be a lot easier than trying to date!" From my friend's point of view, she doesn't understand why it takes Americans so long to make up their minds about choosing a spouse. She often says to me, "Geez, what is the problem? You need five years to decide that you are compatible with a person and could love them? You need to live with them for years to decide? Come on, people know this is going to work long term or it's not. Three months of dating should be plenty of time!" And in a way, she is right. Deep down, most of us know after a few months whether we could marry someone or not. And interestingly, her marriage is one of happiest of all the people I know.

INTRODUCTION

Let's face it. You cannot open a magazine, turn on the TV, hop on the Internet, or talk to friends without the topic of gender differences coming up sooner or later. Communication between men and women is a very popular topic, and self-help books about gender differences top the list of the relationship self-help genre. However, not all communication is gender-related communication. Gender communication is between and about men and women.[1] While sex is simply the biological designation of male or female, "gender is a cultural construction which includes biological sex (male or female), psychological characteristics (femininity, masculinity, androgyny), attitudes about the sexes, and sexual orientation."[2] It is important to learn about the impact of gender roles for many reasons. For example, women are supposed to be nurturing, caring, concerned about the relationship, and better at communicating, but passive. Men are suppose to be dominant in the couple, but stoic, independent, and unconcerned (or less concerned than women) with relationships. Think about the implications of these gender roles. If women are in charge of talking about relationship issues, particularly one as sensitive as sex, yet are also supposed to wait for men to initiate conversations about sex, then it is easy to understand how couples often find themselves at an impasse. Women are more likely to want to talk about sexual issues than men.[3] This could be one reason why talks about sex are so infrequent and uncomfortable between couples. By learning about how gender can affect communication, people can improve their effectiveness as communicators. By better understanding the complex way in which culture affects values and behaviors, people can gain a better insight about their own communication patterns as well as the patterns of the significant others in their lives.

CULTURE AND SEX

It has been said that you never really know your culture until you leave it, until you experience another, very different cultural reality. While in many ways, this is true, it is also true that on several levels, we have an awareness of much of our own culture's characteristics and dynamics. Within this awareness, we know things that we like about our culture as well as things that we don't like about our culture. Despite the fact that we sometimes wish we could change aspects of our own culture, we find ourselves participating in the performance and perpetuation of these very aspects and the associated cultural roles. Cecil Helman defined culture as "a set of guidelines (both explicit and implicit) which individuals inherit as members of a particular society, and which tells them how to view the world, how to experience it emotionally, and how to behave in it in relation to other people."[4] If you reread this definition, you will see that this view of culture does not dismiss social psychology or interpersonal communication. On the contrary, it suggests that culture influences people's interpretations and experiences of life. In the context of sex talk, gender-related dynamics are relevant to whether women will take an active or passive role in sexual situations, including, but not limited to, initiating discussions with a sexual partner about sexual practices and past experiences and using strategies to negotiate or assert power to make their voices understood.

Sexual behavior is symbolic. Humans learn sexuality. As individuals, we learn what kind of sexual creatures we are as we learn gender roles and acquire cultural guidelines regarding such elements of sexuality as desirability, courtship, foreplay, and sexual positions.[5] Humans, no matter the culture, share a universality of having sex. While humans are inherently sexual due to a biological imperative to reproduce, cultural learning directly influences how we go about reproduction: where, when, how often, with whom, and why.[6] The influence of culture on sex cannot be discounted as the "enculturation process is a powerful one, and individuals do not easily cast off its effects."[7] From this viewpoint, culture can be approached as a fundamental component of sex, rather than as a minor influence on sexual behavior. Indeed, "in addition to the fact that we are sexually reproducing creatures is the inescapable fact that sexual reproduction is not the only reason for sexual coupling among humans. Sexual interaction is linked also to play, intimacy, and emotional attachment. These are needs that probably are also a part of our biological makeup as social creatures."[8] Furthermore, we do not necessarily share the same ways across cultures (even within cultures) of enacting, negotiating, and communicating about sex since "these constant and universal features of human sexuality define our capacity in a broad way, but culture shapes the details of local sexual practices around the world."[9]

A cultural context for understanding sexual relationships in general is helpful and useful because it provides "individuals not only with views of how relationships are supposed to develop, but also with vocabularies for representing relationship growth."[10] After all, "interpersonal communication is founded on sociality, on a process that requires shared meaning and awareness of one's accountability to others. All meaningful symbolic engagements within a given culture require that the participants understand together the referents of their discourse and the rules that govern its procedure."[11]

GENDER AND COMMUNICATION

We are born into a sexual category; we are born either male or female. We are socialized into masculine and feminine roles—this aspect is learned. Every society has defined (perhaps loosely or tightly) appropriate gender roles for men and women. Given that gender roles are socially constructed, what is appropriate for the genders has greatly depended on the requirements of a society. For example, people who study feminine and masculine roles describe how in the past, when society was organized around agriculture, the differences between feminine and masculine were less distinct.[12] Both males and females took responsibility for economic survival, cared for children, and overall, there were less distinct divisions of labor. Qualities important in men were emotionality, nurturance, and interdependence, traits essential for agricultural family life. Women were ambitious, strong, and decisive, again essential for success in agricultural-based lives. When the industrial revolution occurred and factories emerged, the working domain of men and women separated, and more modern stereotypical gender differences emerged. For example, the working environment of men was public, utilitarian, and impersonal, while women, who remained at home, became associated with the personal, private, and caregiving activities. These fundamental changes caused the ideals of masculinity to be redefined in terms of independence, aggressiveness, achievement, and self-control. Femininity was redefined as nurturing, relational, and caring for others.[13] We still use these ideals as the basis for many gendered stereotypes today.

NATURE-NURTURE ARGUMENT

Are men and women different based on inherent biological differences (nature) or are they different because they are raised to be different (nurture)? Most people are familiar with the nature-nurture argument. There is evidence to support both sides of this argument. David Lisak, a masculinity researcher, believes that the nature-nurture argument, which explores if gender differences are inherent to a person's sex or if they are learned in society, is false. He contends it is a combination of both nature and nurture. "The nature-nurture argument itself, while seemingly compelling and almost irresistible to engage in, is inherently flawed. If the last twenty years of neuroscience teaches us anything, it is that the brain is a wondrous labyrinth of chemically activated neurocircuitry that is both shaped by genes and constantly altered by environment and experience."[14] This makes the most sense given what we know about biological differences and learned gender behaviors in society. It is safe to conclude that gender differences are a combination of both nature and nurture.

How men and women are "nurtured" into separate gender roles begins at birth. Research has shown that mothers interact differently with male and female babies. Mothers interact more with daughters than sons and keep their daughters physically and psychologically closer. They also tend to be more nurturing with daughters and talk to them more about relationships and personal issues. Mothers have been found to encourage more independence with their sons and to talk to them less about emotional issues and relationships.[15] Some theorists believe this is the reason for differences in how males and females view relationships. Women tend to view relationships as a source of comfort and security, and to affirm self-perceptions as connected with others.[16] However, boys—then men—may view relationships as a threat to their independence.

ARE MEN AND WOMEN THAT DIFFERENT? ARE WE OPPOSITE SEXES?

Most psychologists agree that men and women are much more alike than different. Janet Shibley Hyde, a psychologist who studies gender differences, looked at 46 meta-analyses of studies of psychological gender differences. A meta-analysis is a study that reviews the data from several previous studies on the same topic and tests this larger data set to identify overall trends in a topic. Meta-analyses are considered the most reliable forms of scientific studies. Dr. Shibley Hyde found that "males and females are similar on most, but not all, psychological variables."[17] Ron Levant, a researcher who studies constructs of masculinity, contends that in his review of the available research about gender, that males and females are more alike than different.[18] However, no researcher contends that men and women are constitutionally identical. It recognizes that there are some differences, which can show up in terms of lifestyle, career choices, communication styles, and other differences.

SPEECH COMMUNITIES

Many people are familiar with best-selling self-help books such as *You Just Don't Understand: Women and Men in Conversation,* by Deborah Tannen, and *Men Are from Mars, Women Are from Venus,* by John Gray.[19] While Deborah Tannen, a professor of linguistics at Georgetown College, has much more credibility than John Gray, both have come under scrutiny from scientists and researchers for the claims they make about how men and women communicate. John Gray does not hold any graduate degrees from accredited U.S. schools, nor has his work been reviewed by scholars and leaders in the field of psychology.

Deborah Tannen claims that men and women speak with different styles of communication and that these different styles result in deep-seated misunderstandings between women and men. In other words, men and women use distinctive language codes and draw different inferences from messages. At the heart of her theory is her belief that women use language to include and support others (solidarity), whereas men focus on levels of dominance and control (power) in communicative interactions. The problem with Tannen's (and Gray's) approach to gender is that they view gender as one-dimensional in the sense that women and men are presented as fundamentally different. They speak different languages and reason differently. As we see in this chapter, although we can draw some conclusions based on gender, gender is unique to all individuals and ever changing because we are constantly evolving as people in any give time or culture. Renowned gender and communication researcher and professor at the University of North Carolina, Chapel Hill, Julia Wood has written an excellent text titled *Gendered Lives.* Many of the examples I use in this chapter are discussed in her book. One important concept Julia Wood researched and presented is that of gendered speech communities; that is, there are feminine and masculine styles of verbal communication. Wood expands on the 1982 classic study completed by Daniel Maltz and Ruth Borker, who studied games that children play and how they cultivate different methods of communication. Specifically, Wood explained that games such as baseball and soccer are formative tools in how males develop communication patterns. First, look at the kinds of games boys play. They often involve large groups; they are competitive in nature, goal oriented, have winners and losers, involve physically rough play, and often have a set of rules and specific roles or positions. Wood asserts that boys' games promote basic communication rules:

1. Boys use communication to assert ideas, opinions, and identity.
2. Boys use communication to achieve something such as problem solving or strategy development.
3. Boys use communication to attract and maintain attention.
4. Boys communicate to compete for the "talk stage." Boys talk to stand out, take attention away from others, and gain attention from others.[20]

Although many young people deny that there are still significant differences between boys and girls, research shows that differences still exist. For example, most elementary school–aged children prefer same-sex playmates. Overall, boys use communication to compete with one another, exert control over others, and accomplish goals, all of which are focused on individuality, competition, and achievement. Interestingly, grown men still tend to do things with their friends, rather than build and maintain relationships through talk.

Think about the messages we send to little boys: "don't cry," "don't be a sissy," "play hard, take chances, winning is important," "you are so strong, such a big boy," "stand up for yourself." Boys are praised for strength, independence, and achievements. Now think about what this means for how boys are taught to communicate. They are taught to be dominant, to voice their opinions, to be leaders and say what they think. Other traditional qualities associated with masculinity are toughness, self-reliance, and invulnerability. Boys learn that to be popular in elementary school, they need to be aggressive and good at sports. Girls in elementary school learn that popular girls are kind, pretty, and have pretty clothes.

What about girls? Girls tend to play in small groups or pairs and rarely play organized games; rather, games such as "house" or "school" rarely have formal rules, do not have winners and losers, and most of the time, girls talk to each other as the game progresses to make up or change the game. While playing, girls spend more time talking than doing anything else, thus developing their interpersonal communication skills. In the end, Julia Wood contended that girls learn the following rules of communication from the games they play:

1. Girls use communication to create and maintain relationships. The focus is on the process of communication and not the content of what is being said.
2. Girls use communication to establish egalitarian relationships with others. They do not use communication to criticize, put down, or outdo others.
3. Girls use communication to include others. They attempt to bring others into conversations and talk about their ideas.
4. Girls use communication to show sensitivity and value relationships. We can see that girls focus on cooperation and open-ended processes.[21]

Think about the messages we teach little girls: "share with others, don't be selfish," "be careful, you don't want to hurt yourself," "don't get too dirty," "be gentle," "be polite." Girls are praised for helping others, playing house, looking pretty, and being neat, smart, and sweet. Now think about what this means for how girls are taught to communicate. They are taught to listen to and appreciate what others are saying, not to interrupt others, and to be patient and kind when communicating.

DIFFERENCES IN HOW MEN AND WOMEN COMMUNICATE

Many communication scholars believe that men and women differ on what they believe to be the function of communication.[22] Although this is a generalization, men approach conversations to impart information (called the content aspect of communication) rather than to convey cues about the relationship (called the relational aspect of communication). Women tend to converse more as an indication of the relationship rather than to impart information. Therefore men tend to use communication for information exchange rather than for relationship development. We can see some evidence of this in the way men and women form same-sex friendships. Men tend to do things with their friends, while women tend to maintain their friendships through talk. One of my communication studies professors liked to tell a story about one of his closest friends. They were next-door neighbors and jogged together four times a week for 10 years. They usually carried on a conversation during parts of their run and always during their cool-down walk. One morning, my professor asked his friend, "So, how is your wife doing these days?" His friend responded by saying, "We separated three months ago." He was floored. My professor considered himself to be an excellent communicator and nurturing friend; after all, he had a PhD in communication, was the dean of the college of communication, and had taught interpersonal communication for over 30 years. He was shocked that his friend did not mention that he was having marital difficulties, let alone that he had separated from his wife. My professor often used this example when teaching about gender differences to highlight how men communicate (or fail to communicate) with one another.

Women tend to use communication to establish and maintain relationships with other people. We can see that women often communicate to maintain relationships with others, mainly by inquiring about a person. Women often ask questions such as "How was your day?"

"How are you feeling?" "Anything interesting happen today at work?" It is important for women to establish equality with others, creating an interactive process of communication, taking talk turns with others in the conversation. Women tend to use communication to provide support for one another by asking many questions and providing sympathetic comments. Feminine communication is often very personal; women share stories about themselves and their lives, disclosing personal information. Women rarely use direct commands or make direct comments. Researchers have found that women use tag questions and verbal hedges significantly more than men. Tag questions are questions at the end of a statement such as "That was an interesting movie, wasn't it?" "I am so annoyed we have to wait this long, aren't you?" Hedges are tentative statements such as "I think that he might not be happy with our project" or "I feel like maybe you don't want to go to dinner tonight." It is a softer way of communicating, although sometimes men get frustrated with hedges. Men who prefer direct communication styles tend to be annoyed by hedges and tag questions and say they would rather women simply tell them what they want or think.

According to Julia Wood and her thorough examination of research about gender and communication, men tend to avoid personal disclosures when communicating; rather, they communicate to accomplish goals, gain control, maintain independence, entertain, and gain status. Talk is a way to prove themselves, and sometimes men even see winners and losers in conversations. How many times have you heard a man say "I won that round," and I imagine that woman might be thinking, "It was just a conversation; I didn't know it was a competition." Research has also shown that men tend to give advice when communicating. This is a way for them to exhibit knowledge and take control. Because masculine communication is focused on problem solving, talk is focused on getting information, uncovering facts, and then suggesting solutions. Talk is informational. Interestingly, men talk at greater length and more often than women. This is not limited to face-to-face conversations; in fact, men talk longer and more often than women in Internet conversations and in e-mail discussion groups. Men also tend to interrupt more than women. Masculine talk is direct and assertive and tends to be less emotionally responsive. Men give what are called minimum response cues such as "yeah" or "um." The differences between how men and women communicate affect their approaches to sex talk. In some ways, these differences limit communication between couples, but by understanding these differences and identifying the ones most prevalent in your relationships, you can address them and hopefully overcome them.

ATTRACTION, LOVE, ROMANCE, AND SEX: GENDER DIFFERENCES

Elizabeth McGee of the University of California, San Diego and Mark Shelvin reviewed what men and women find attractive in a mate.[23] Their research showed that men value physical attractiveness and youth in a partner more than women. They concluded that women value characteristics in men such as dependability, good earning capacity, ambition, a career-oriented mentality, and high socioeconomic status. I do not think anyone would be surprised by these results. However, other psychologists who reviewed findings from various studies generally indicate that intrinsic attributes (e.g., honesty, kindness, dependability) are relatively more important for a long-term relationship, whereas external attributes (e.g., physical appearance such as attractiveness) are more important for a short-term relationship.[24]

Interestingly, McGee and Shelvin found that both men and women value a good sense of humor in a potential life partner. One reason humor is so highly valued is that it implies the presence of other positive traits such as pleasantness. In fact, McGee and Shelvin found that people described as being well above average in sense of humor were seen as lower in neuroticism and higher in agreeableness than individuals described as typical or below average in terms of sense of humor. Additionally, individuals with higher humor orientation were associated with lower levels of loneliness and were viewed as socially attractive.

Although a popular belief in society is that women are more concerned with romance and are more romantic than men, research shows that in general, men are more romantic than women. Men tend to fall in love harder and faster than women. Men play more games than women. Men are more active, sexualized, impulsive, and spontaneous than women. Men and women also differ on definitions of romance and intimacy. Jane Ridely,[25] a psychiatrist and couples counselor, agreed that men and women define intimacy differently. Whereas women do not see sex as a necessary or integral part of intimacy, men do. Men enjoy romantic gestures such as spontaneous love making, excursions to romantic places, and surprising women with gifts and flowers. Women tend to see romantic relationships as deep friendships and, on the whole, are more pragmatic than men when it comes to romance. Women find deep conversations, intimacy (not necessarily sexual), and the sharing of feelings to be romantic. Thus some men see sex as an essential component to intimacy, whereas some women do not. When men talk about sex, the approach necessarily includes sex as a desired outcome, whereas women may see the talk itself as an intimate act.

DIFFERENCES IN MALE AND FEMALE SEXUALITY

Renowned psychologist and sexuality expert Letitia Anne Peplau believes that there are four main differences in male and female sexuality. In her aptly titled article "Human Sexuality: How Do Men and Women Differ?" Peplau explains the four distinctions:

First, on a wide variety of measures, men show greater sexual desire than do women. Second, compared with men, women place greater emphasis on committed relationships as a context for sexuality. Third, aggression is more strongly linked to sexuality for men than for women. Fourth, women's sexuality tends to be more malleable and capable of change over time. These male-female differences are pervasive, affecting thoughts and feelings as well as behavior, and they characterize not only heterosexuals but lesbians and gay men as well.[26]

As Peplau further explains in her article, although men and women are more similar than different when it comes to sexuality, these differences are important to recognize. First, Peplau defines the term *sexual desire* as an interest in sexual objects and activities and the wish to partake in sexual activity. Across the life span, men report higher levels of sex drive than women. Numerous research reports indicate that men also desire greater frequency of sex and that for most heterosexual couples, the frequency of sex is often a compromise between men and women. This is interesting given the statistics about sexual activity in chapter one, in particular the fact that current research also shows that men are more likely than women to stop having sex in long term relationships. When one member desires less sex and that person is the man, then couples tend to stop having sex. One reason for this could be the idea that men really are more in control of sexual activities in heterosexual relationships.

Second, there are significant differences between men and women and the role of relationships in sexual activity. Women view committed relationships as a context for sex, while men easily separate sex from romance and commitment. There are clear ramifications for many young women who hope for a close, romantic relationship after a casual sexual encounter and are disappointed when men do not respond in kind. Third, in a review of research that investigated the sexual self-concepts of men and women, both genders showed dimensions of romance and passion; however, men's self-concepts also included aggression. In terms of sexuality, men saw themselves as aggressive, powerful, experienced, domineering, and individualistic. Women did not see themselves this way. Researchers concluded that aggression is closely linked to sexuality for men, yet not women. The last concept that Peplau discussed was sexual plasticity, the level of influence that cultural, social, and situational factors can have on sexuality. Each of these four issues is discussed in greater detail in the following paragraphs.

In terms of male sexuality, one of the most common scales to measure the level of "masculinity" among men is called the Male Role Norms Inventory. This inventory or scale is used to determine the characteristics of masculinity. Unfortunately, high levels of masculinity were found to be linked to a range of problematic individual and relational variables. Some of these troubling indicators included a reluctance to "discuss condom use with partners, fear of intimacy, lower relationship satisfaction . . . self reports of sexual aggression, lower forgiveness of racial discrimination, alexithymia (the inability to express feelings with words) and related constructs, and reluctance to seek psychological help."[27] Too much masculinity is not a good thing for quality communication.

Sexual identity is "the enduring sense of oneself as a sexual being which fits a culturally created category and accounts for one's sexual fantasies, attractions, and behaviors."[28] Sexual identity for women is not just based on sexual feelings and behaviors; rather, because women view sex as a way to establish intimacy and maintain close personal relationships, sexual identity is linked to romance and not just sex. The fact that in American culture, we place so much more emphasis on sex than relationships in our society could be because of male domination of media, relationships, communication in relationships, and so forth. If women were in power positions, we might see a greater emphasis on relational issues, but one cannot be positive.

Social psychologists believe that female sexuality is more fluid and flexible than male sexuality. In other words, female sexuality is malleable and capable of change over time, whereas male sexuality is believed to be rooted in biology and childhood experiences.[29] In 2000, psychologist Roy Baumeister came up with the idea of measuring gender differences in what he calls *erotic plasticity*.[30] Plasticity is the degree to which a person's sex drive can be formed and changed by cultural, social, and situational pressures. So, if a person has limited erotic plasticity, then Baumeister contends that that person's sexuality is firmly formed in early life, either though biological determinants or through childhood experiences. Baumeister presents compelling evidence in the scientific paper he wrote that women have more erotic plasticity because education, religion, and culture have a greater impact on women's sexu-ality than on men's sexuality. This is in part due to the fact that women's sexuality is more complex and emotional than that of men. Women are more likely to romanticize sexual desire—considering the act of sex as something to establish emotional intimacy and express love for another person—whereas men are more likely to sexualize desire; to men, sex is physical and desire is the physical wanting of someone.[31] Most psychologists believe that women have a partner-centered or relational approach to sex, while men tend to think of sex as recreation and body centered.[32] This is not to say that eroticism and sex are not important to women or that emotional intimacy is not important to men; it is simply to say that it is important to acknowledge the role that emotional intimacy has on women's sexual experiences and communication about sex. For example, if emotional intimacy is important to a woman's sexual experiences, communication with her partner is essential to establishing and maintaining a quality sex life.

Do men and women think about sex differently? Yes, according to sex researchers Susan Sprecher and Kathleen McKinney.[33] In a review of a large number of scientific articles, they concluded that men have a more positive attitude toward sex, toward premarital sex, casual sex, and multiple sexual partners. And it is true that men also think about sex a lot more than women—for men, the end goal of sex is physical gratification—and indicate that partner initiative and variety of sexual activities are important to them. Therefore it makes sense that men see more women as potential sexual partners (men are less discriminating) than women see men as sexual partners.

Ellis and Symons contend that even women's sexual fantasies are different from those of men.[34] More often, women's fantasies include a partner who they know, include affection and communication, and describe a setting for the sexual activity. In contrast, men's fantasies more often involve multiple partners, strangers, and anonymous partners and are focused on specific sexual acts and sexual organs.

SEXUAL DOUBLE STANDARDS: DO THEY EXIST, AND IF SO, TO WHAT EXTENT?

A sexual double standard is the belief that men are praised for sexual activity, whereas women are penalized.[35] In other words, men are rewarded socially for sexual exploits, and women are socially derogated for the same behaviors.[36] And while men are valued for their sexual promiscuity, women are not. Within gender roles, it is expected that women are innocent, men experienced. This is apparent in the double standard that compels men to feel as if they should lose their virginity as soon as possible and for women to maintain it as long as possible. Due to the fact that many women are expected to be both virgins and have sex, this places them in a paradox. "The expression of female desire, then, can be a risky enterprise for young women. The sexual double standard is regulated through the tool of sexual reputation, which is the negative labeling of an active, desiring female sexuality and positive labeling of active male sexuality."[37] Having to negotiate these fine boundaries is one of the reasons why communication about sex is so complicated.

Michael Marks and Chris Fraley set out to review the empirical research on the actual presence of the sexual double standard in U.S. society in their scholarly article "The Sexual Double Standard: Fact or Fiction?" While they cite research that showed that the "sexual double standard seems to be a ubiquitous phenomenon in contemporary society; one recent survey revealed that 85% of people believe that a double standard exists in our culture."[38] In their research, they had people read vignettes of males and females who were described as sexually promiscuous or having a limited number of partners. Both males and females were rated lower in terms of likeability, morality, and desirability as a spouse when they rated the people who had a high number of sexual partners. In a review of literature and their own study, they found that for people who had high numbers of sexual partners, both male and female were viewed negatively by participants. They suggest that instead of people researching the double standard, people need to address why the false double standard belief is so pervasive. Indeed, expectations of chastity and virginity have been steadily declining in the United States since the 1950s. In a series of repeated tests beginning in the early 1940s, men and women were given a list of 18 attributes that they were looking for in a mate and to rate them in terms of importance. Chastity, the lack of sexual experience, was one of the attributes and, in 1945, was ranked 10th in terms of importance. The exact same test was repeated in 1969, and virginity had fallen to 15th in terms of importance in a mate. The year 1981 was the last time the study was done, and men ranked chastity in a partner at 18th out of 18 constructs—dead last in terms of importance.[39] Clearly the importance of sexual experience and chastity is culturally determined. In some Asian countries, sexual inexperience (even virginity) of women is considered attractive by men. In some Western European countries, such as France, Sweden, and Italy, sexual inexperience is viewed negatively for both men and women.

IMPLICATIONS FOR SEX TALK

We learned in this chapter that men are supposed to be highly sexual. This means that they are supposed to be interested in sex all the time, any time. They are expected to be sexually experienced, and the more partners that a man has, the better. This is one area that men talk about with one another—sexual conquests. Men frequently joke about sex with one another, as well. Boys learn at a young age that they are supposed to have lots of girlfriends; one of the participants in my study about communication about sex said that he was often asked by his father, "How many girlfriends are you going to have when you grow up?" He reported that his sisters were never asked how many boyfriends they were going to have when they grew up. One thing that men learn more than anything else is that a cornerstone of masculinity is not to be feminine: "don't be such a girl," "you throw like a girl," "don't be a crybaby," "what a mama's boy," "you are pussy whipped," "she wears the pants in your relationship," "what do you mean you don't want to have sex?" Both men and women often ridicule men who engage in these behaviors. So men learn "not to be like girls," yet women expect them to be supportive, caring, open, romantic, emotional, and to fully take part in raising children and taking care of the house. This is a difficult dilemma for men. Interestingly, women tend to enforce these gender roles just as much as other men. Men are often afraid to let themselves go in front of women because they fear the consequences.

Men and women even talk about their sexual experiences differently, which is reflected by male sexual aggression and female submission. When men have sex, particularly with a new partner, they use words and expressions like "I scored." This implies that there was a great deal of effort involved, physical prowess, and something to be proud of, just like on the playing field, where people literally score. It's a good thing to score. Women rarely say things like "I scored." Even on shows like *Sex and the City*, the female characters often describe sexual activity as "we did the deed" or "it just happened." Women frequently describe their sexual experiences, particularly young women and women who are involved in casual sexual experiences, as "it just happened." This indicates that they have clearly learned the gender role of female sexual passivity and most likely believe that sex really did "just happen." It implies that women did not make a conscious decision to have sex or admit (even to themselves) that they have sexual desires, let alone actively pursue sex and "score." Not only is it acceptable for men to admit that they have strong sexual desires, but it is expected.

Psychologists Amy Kiefer and Diana Sanchez believe that gender roles decrease sexual function and satisfaction. They believe that sexual autonomy is a requirement for both men and women to enjoy sex and that gender roles limit sexual autonomy. We know that sexual satisfaction is important for relational happiness, duration, and success. Kiefer and Sanchez strongly believe that for women, in particular, adherence to traditional gender-based sexual roles can significantly hinder the development of an enjoyable and satisfying sexual relationship for both partners. However, for women to let go of learned sex roles and scripts for how they are supposed to behave in bed is not easy. In the end, women are still held responsible for the consequences of sexual activity. Social mores in the United States require that women take more responsibility than men.[40] Ultimately, both men and women believe that women would be responsible for any consequences of sex and therefore should be responsible for birth control and ensuring condom use.[41] While there have been cultural changes about accepting women's sexuality and a more liberal approach to multiple partners, cultural gender roles necessitate women's silence about their personal sexual experiences. In other words, they have the opportunity for more sexual experiences but are in many ways denied the opportunity to communicate in meaningful ways about those experiences. This silence limits their ability not only to be open about their own sexual histories and current practices, but also to have discussions about their partners' sexual histories and current practices.

Women are often constrained in their communication about sex because their traditional gender roles indicate that they should wait for a man to bring up the topic. Also, they may be afraid that a man might get mad if he thinks she is somehow unhappy with their sex life. More often, women do not want to hurt their partners' feelings or offend their partners' manhood; after all, men are supposed to be highly sexual and to be really "good in bed." In a study I conducted about male and female communication about sex, most female participants reported that they did not talk about sex with their partners; they preferred to talk about their sexual experiences or relationships with close friends. This makes sense knowing what we do about feminine communication styles. However, talking with your best friend about sex probably will not help your sex life (although it might make you feel better). In my opening story, Krissy has not had sex with her husband in two years, since her twins were born. She talks about it once in a while with Sue but never broaches the topic with her husband. Why not?

While each gender is socialized into different roles and communication patterns, neither gender is really taught how, when, or why to talk about sex. This is one area that we neglect as a society. If people feel they will be ridiculed or rejected for initiating meaningful, serious discussion about sex, it is easy to see why more of these conversations do not take place.

Recall that humans, no matter the culture, share a universality of having sex, but there are significant relational—thus cultural and gendered—differences that influence how and why people have sex, and in extension, how and why people communicate about sex. So while society sometimes likes to frame sex in strictly biological or medical terms, it should not ignore the very human and communication-based needs that go along with sexual relationships such as intimacy and emotional attachment.

Also, because women link sex with relationships, they are more likely to comply with unwanted sexual advances than men. If a wife is not in the mood, she may go ahead and have sex so as not to hurt her husband's feelings and preserve the relationship. Because men have a more physical view of sex, rather than relational, they are less likely to comply with sexual overtures if they are not in the mood. In turn, women may see this as a personal attack rather than a physical unwillingness.

In this chapter, I offered readers peer-reviewed research from accredited sources about theories and hypotheses that have been studied in a systematic way, rather than offering kitschy anecdotal observations about men and women. I do not claim that such self-help books are completely inaccurate about the information and observations they make. Indeed, it does not take a PhD or an MD to discern some basic truths about men and women. However, I would like readers to keep in mind that overwhelming evidence supports that men and women are much more alike physiologically and psychologically than they are different. I offer you this explanatory paragraph because some of the findings I present in this chapter about how men and women communicate both echo some of the claims in popular self-help books and repudiate others. Ultimately, the focus of this chapter is to help the reader understand how gender and culture affect sexual communication.

NOTES

1. Diana Ivy and Phil Backlund, *Genderspeak: Personal Effectiveness in Gender Communication* (Boston: McGraw-Hill, 2004).

2. Ibid., 34.

3. Mike Allen, Tara M. Emmers-Sommer, and Tara L. Crowell, "Couples Negotiating Safer Sex Behaviors: A Meta-Analysis of the Impact of Conversation and Gender," in *Interpersonal Communication Research: Advances through Meta-Analysis*, ed. Raymond W. Preiss, Barbara Mae Gayle, and Nancy A. Burrell (Mahwah, NJ: Lawrence Erlbaum Associates, 2002), 273.

4. Cecil Helman, *Culture, Health and Illness*, 2nd ed. (London: Wright, 1990), 2–3.

5. DeWight Middleton, *Exotics and Erotics: Human Cultural and Sexual Diversity* (Prospect Heights, IL: Waveland, 2002).

6. Michael Kimmel and Jeffrey Fracher, "Hard Issues and Soft Spots: Counseling Men about Sexuality," in *Men's Lives*, ed. Michael Kimmel and Michael Messner (New York: Macmillan, 1992).

7. Robert Middleton and Edward Laumann, "Introduction: Setting the Scene," in *Sex, Love, and Health in America: Private Choices and Public Policies*, ed. Robert Middleton and Edward Laumann (Chicago: University of Chicago Press, 2002), 38.

8. Ibid., 26.

9. Ibid.

10. Steve Duck, Linda West, and L. K Acitelli, "Sewing the Field: The Tapestry of Relationships in Life and Research," in *Handbook of Personal Relationships*, ed. Steve Duck (Chichester, NY: John Wiley, 1997), 15.

11. Walter J. Carl and Steve Duck, "How to Do Things with Relationships . . . and How Relationships Do Things with Us," in *Communication Yearbook*, ed. Pamela Kalbfleisch (Mahwah, NJ: Lawrence Erlbaum Associates, 2004), 12.

12. Francesca Cancian, "Love and the Rise of Capitalism," in *Gender in Intimate Relationships: A Micro Structural Approach*, ed. Barbara Riseman and Pepper Schwartz (Belmont, CA: Wadsworth, 1989).

13. Ibid.

14. David Lisak, 2006, http://SPSMM@Lists.apa.org (Accessed July 6, 2006).

15. Judith Lorber, *Gender Inequality: Feminist Theories and Politics*, 2nd ed. (Los Angeles, CA: Roxbury Press, 2001).

16. Julia Wood, *Gendered Lives*, 7th ed. (Belmont, CA: Thompson Wadsworth, 2007).

17. Janet Shibley Hyde, "The Gender Similarities Hypothesis," *American Psychologist* 60, no. 6 (2005): 581.

18. Ronald F. Levant and Katherine Richmond, "A Review of Research on Masculinity Ideologies Using the Male Role Norms Inventory," *Journal of Men's Studies* 15 (2007): 130–46.

19. John Gray, *Men Are from Mars, Women Are from Venus* (New York: HarperCollins, 1992). Deborah Tannen, *You Just Don't Understand: Women and Men in Conversation* (New York: Morrow, 1990).

20. Wood, *Gendered Lives*, 124–25.

21. Julia Wood, *But I Thought You Meant . . . Misunderstandings in Human Communication* (Mountain View, CA: Mayfield, 1998). The reference for the original study can be found in Daniel Maltz and Ruth Borker, "A Cultural Approach to Male-Female Miscommunication," in John Gumpert, ed., *Language and Social Identity* (Cambridge: Cambridge University Press, 1982), 196–216.

22. Paul Watzlawick, Janet Beavin, and Don Jackson, *Pragmatics of Human Communication* (New York: W. W. Norton, 1967). Wood, *But I Thought You Meant*.

23. Elizabeth McGee and Mark Shevlin, "Effect of Humor on Interpersonal Attraction and Mate Selection," *Journal of Psychology* 143 (2009).

24. Douglas T. Kenrick, Edward K. Sadalla, Gary Groth, and Melanie R. Trost, "Evolution, Traits, and the Stages of Human Courtship: Qualifying the Parental Investment Model," *Journal of Personality* 58 (1990). Pamela C. Regan and Ellen Berscheid, "Gender Differences in Characteristics Desired in a Potential Sexual and Marriage Partner," *Journal of Psychology and Human Sexuality* 9, no. 1 (1997).

25. Jane Ridely, "Gender and Couples: Do Men and Women Seek Different Kinds of Intimacy?" *Sexual and Marital Therapy* 8, no. 3 (1993).

26. Letitia Anne Peplau, "Human Sexuality: How Do Men and Women Differ?" *Current Directions in Psychological Science* 12, no. 2 (2003): 37.

27. Levant and Richmond, "A Review of Research," 142.

28. Ritch Savin-Williams, "Lesbian, Gay Male and Bisexual Adolescents," in *Lesbian, Gay, and Bisexual Identities over the Lifespan*, ed. Anthony D'Augelli and C. J. Patternson (New York: Oxford University Press, 1995), 165–89.

29. Letitia Anne Peplau and Linda D. Garnets, "A New Paradigm for Understanding Women's Sexuality and Sexual Orientation," *Journal of Social Issues* 56, no. 2 (2000).

30. Roy F. Baumeister, "Gender Differences in Erotic Plasticity: The Female Sex Drive as Socially Flexible and Responsive," *Psychological Bulletin* 126, no. 3 (2000).

31. Regan and Berscheid, "Gender Differences in Characteristics Desired."

32. Janet Shibley Hyde and John D. DeLamater, *Understanding Human Sexuality*, 7th ed. (New York: McGraw-Hill, 2000).

33. Susan Sprecher and Kathleen McKinney, *Sexuality* (Newbury Park, CA: Sage, 1993).

34. Bruce J. Ellis and Donald Symons, "Sex Differences in Sexual Fantasy: An Evolutionary Psychological Approach," *Journal of Sex Research* 27, no. 4 (1990).

35. Kathryn Greene and Sandra Faulkner, "Gender, Belief in the Sexual Double Standard, and Sexual Talk in Heterosexual Dating Relationships," *Sex Roles* 53 (2005).

36. Michael J. Marks and R. Chris Fraley, "The Sexual Double Standard: Fact or Fiction?" *Sex Roles* 52 (2005).

37. Susan Jackson and Fiona Cram, "Disrupting the Sexual Double Standard: Young Women's Talk about Heterosexuality," *British Journal of Social Psychology* 42, Pt. 1 (2003): 114.

38. Marks and Fraley, "Sexual Double Standard," 175. Michael Marks, "Internet Survey of Attitudes of Sexual Freedom," unpublished raw data, 2002. Robin Milhausen and Edward Herold, "Reconceptualizing the Sexual Double Standard," *Journal of Psychology and Human Sexuality* 13, no. 63–83 (2001). Robin Milhausen and Edward Herold, "Does the Sexual Double Standard Still Exist? Perceptions of University Women," *Journal of Sex Research* 36 (1999).

39. Pamela Regan, *The Dating Game*, 2nd ed. (Thousand Oaks, CA: Sage, 2008). Complete review on pp. 190–92.

40. Allen et al., "Couples Negotiating Safer Sex Behaviors," 273.

41. Carey M. Noland, "Listening to the Sound of Silence: Gender Roles and Communication about Sex in Puerto Rico," *Sex Roles* 55, no. 5 (2006).

CHAPTER 4

Getting to the Heart of the Matter: The Importance of Nonverbal Communication in Sexual Relationships

"Do you see that woman in the blue dress with her friends over there? She wants me," Joe said to his friends. It was a Friday night in the summer, and everyone was out at the beach having a good time. Joe's friends did not take him too seriously as Joe thought women always wanted him and, in their opinion, he was rarely correct. It was even more rare that he ever got a phone number because he never had enough nerve to actually go up and talk to the women he thought wanted him.

"OK, Joe, why don't you explain this revelation to us. How do you know that woman in the blue dress wants you?" Billy, a guy in the group who always went home with the most phone numbers in his pocket, asked.

"Well, it's obvious to the trained eye. She keeps looking over at us and her gaze lingers on me. She flips her hair when she looks at me and kind of smiles. It's the classic female sign of 'I want you,'" Joe reported with confidence.

"Ha, the door is behind us, you idiot. She could be looking for a friend coming in or just checking out the new men as they walk in. You are standing directly in front of the door. She cannot not look at you."

"No, it's me she is looking at, her gaze lingers, man. I am telling you," Joe insisted.

"OK, then go up to her and talk to her. Let's see how interested she really is," one of his friends taunted him.

"No, if she wants me, she should come to me. She will, if she wants me enough and nobody else better looking than me hits on her before closing time."

"Yeah, let's just see, Joe, let's just see." One of his friends decided to let him off the hook because he could see Joe was becoming uncomfortable.

In reality, Joe is not that far off the mark. He did read the nonverbal signs correctly, if indeed the woman in the blue dress was looking at him and not at the door. So much of what men and women do in courtship and sexual relationships is guided by nonverbal cues that it would be impossible to measure and count the impact of each cue. However, this chapter does provide insight into much of what goes on in terms of nonverbal communication and sex.

INTRODUCTION

Understanding nonverbal communication is particularly important when learning how to talk about sex because so much of how people communicate about sex is nonverbal. Research has shown that is it actually much easier and more comfortable for people to have sex than to talk about it, particularly at the beginning of a romantic relationship.[1] In my research on communication about sex, when asked about how either women or men could and do initiate sex, I learned that such efforts of sexual advancement were primarily nonverbal in nature. Touch, physical proximity and contact, hints, location, and other nonverbal cues such as buying dinner or drinks, the way you dress, flirting, body movement, dancing in a certain way, and so on, are ways people let others know they want to have sex with them. However, as nonverbal symbols, none of these messages are conclusive indications that a person wants sex or wants to have sex with you. Certainly relying on nonverbal symbols to do your talking for you, to get your message across, is an ambiguous and indirect form of communication, one that often leads directly to misunderstandings. And yet, this is how so many people begin and maintain sexual relationships.

These sentiments support other research that shows that sexual encounters, at least early in a relationship, often involve very little spoken communication; rather, communication is nonverbal and coded. I believe that there is a very specific and functional reason for this. Ambiguity is deliberately maintained in case one of the partners decides not to proceed. With the risk that is involved with an offer of sex, rejection is a very real possibility; people are interested in minimizing this risk, accomplished through maintaining ambiguity. Even when communication of sexual initiation turned verbal, it was often only a suggestive whisper.

Reliance on nonverbal communication is not limited to those dating; many married couples rely on nonverbal cues to let their partner know they want to have sex. People may play a certain kind of music, light candles, wear certain clothing, or open a bottle of wine to let their spouse know, "Hey, I want to have sex, do you?" Married couples know what these signs are—candles mean romance and/or sex. This lets us avoid direct dialogue involved in initiating sex—"hey, do you want to do it?" or "do you want to make love?"—that forces people to admit that they want sex and risk outright verbal rejection. When presented with nonverbal sex cues, a partner can choose either to have sex or decline, but in a way that allows the other person to save face. If a person is not interested in sex, he can offer a variety of reasons that have nothing to do with the person: "oh, candles . . . I had a really long day at the office and my back is killing me, but they are so nice to look at. Thanks for lighting them." He can let his wife know that sex is out, but let's pretend that you put the candles out for ambiance. It might seem surprising that married couples, even after years of marriage, are reluctant to make blatant sexual overtures toward their partners, but there are many reasons why this might happen, and getting rejected, even by a spouse, still hurts. If a person gets rejected enough, then she might eventually stop asking, which is one reason why so many couples are in sexless marriages.

OVERVIEW OF NONVERBAL COMMUNICATION

In the area of communication studies, researchers place a high level of importance on nonverbal communication in face-to-face interactions. People decode both verbal and nonverbal meanings from an interaction but place most of the interpretation—up to 65 percent of it—on the nonverbal cues that accompany and surround that verbal message. People also tend to perceive that nonverbal messages are more truthful, partly because it's harder to hide a facial expression than to form appropriate word responses. Also, many nonverbal actions may be unintentional and reactive—a raised voice in anger or a smile at a joke—something that we have less control over than spoken words. As a culture, we know that there are different meanings for nonverbal cues, even something like a smile. A smile generally conveys happiness or pleasure, but it could also be used as a way to save face or admit guilt in an uncomfortable situation.

Nonverbal communication consists of the bodily actions and vocal qualities that accompany verbal messages. Bodily actions include eye contact, gestures, and posture. Eye contact is of particular importance in sexual relationships for obvious reasons. While the amount of eye contact can vary from person to person, studies show that talkers hold eye contact 40 percent of the time, while listeners maintain it nearly 70 percent of the time.[2] In general, people tend to make more eye contact when discussing subjects that they are comfortable with, that they are interested in, or when they are trying to be persuasive. Likewise, when topics are embarrassing, when we have something to hide, or when we are ashamed, we tend to avoid eye contact. Women tend to have more frequent eye contact than men and hold the eye contact for longer periods.[3] When communicating with people about sex, it is valuable to remember the importance of eye contact. You may be able to tell how embarrassed or ashamed someone is by his nonverbal cues and, in particular, his eye contact or lack of eye contact. However, it is important to remember that research has also shown that people avoid eye contact when they want to afford someone privacy.[4] This most often happens in public places, for example, a couple is arguing on a bus and you turn your eyes away as if to say, "I am giving you privacy as best I can. I do not want to intrude." So a man might avoid eye contact with his teenage child when discussing sexual education to give her some level of privacy and distance in the conversation.

Another important form of nonverbal communication in regard to sex is touch. Touch communication is known as *haptics* and is thought to be the most primitive form of communication. For humans, it is probably the first sense to be used, even in the womb. People who know and care about each other and who are in an intimate relationship expect touch frequently and assess touch positively. Research has demonstrated that people are more receptive to and evaluate touch as more desirable when the communicator is physically attractive. Furthermore, different types of touch convey different types of meanings. For example, among a pat, a stroke, a squeeze, and a brush, a pat is seen as the most "playful and friendly" and a stroke as the most "loving, pleasant and sexual."[5] Researchers Stanley Jones and Elaine Yarbrough identified five major meanings that touch communicates.[6] Some of these are positive emotions, including support, appreciation, inclusion, sexual interest or intent, and affection. Couples touch the most in the intermediate stage of their relationships, more so than at the beginning or in firmly established relationships.[7] Women initiate more opposite sex touching—especially opposite sex touching that is designed to control. These touching behaviors might indicate "move over," "hurry," or "do it." Interestingly, touch has also been found to facilitate self-disclosure.[8] Women initiate touch more in married relationships and less in casual dating relationships than do men.[9] Opposite sex friends report more touching than same-sex friends. This is probably due to societal norms against same-sex touching, particularly for men.

It is widely accepted that touch is important to us as humans. Recent research shows the value of touch for infants. In a study at the School of Medicine at the University of Miami, doctors showed that premature babies grow faster and gain more weight when massaged.[10] Researchers found that premature babies who are massaged three times a day have 47 percent more weight gain than those who are not massaged. Appropriate touching has been shown to increase liking and compliance. In experiments where people were asked to do something, they complied significantly more often when the request was accompanied by a brief touch on the arm. For example, in one study by professors Gueguen and Fischer-LoKou, "undercover" people who worked for the professors asked people walking by on the street to look after their large and hyperactive dog for 10 minutes while they went into a pharmacy that did not allow dogs.[11] When the undercover researcher touched the person lightly and asked for the favor, it worked 55 percent of the time. When the undercover researcher did not touch people and asked in the exact same way, only 35 percent of the people agreed. This is a significant difference and demonstrates that touching, even among strangers, can be persuasive. The amount of touching we experience decreases with age, and studies have shown that older men are particularly uncomfortable being touched by women compared to other segments of the population.

It is clear how touch and even eye contact (a look) manifest as replacements for verbal communication when it comes to sex talk about things such as expectations or desires during sex. It is much easier to touch someone a certain way or to grab her hand and it put somewhere or to use vocal cues (a moan) to let your partner know what you want. Nonverbal communication is an important part of communicating about sex—especially when communicating during sex—however, it should not be the only way we communicate with our partners. We should try to have direct verbal communication about sexual likes and dislikes so there is limited ambiguity regarding this important area of our lives. Conversations about sex do not need to be during or even after sexual intercourse, but people should find some agreed upon time that works for both people to discuss important matters.

You can increase the amount that you and your sexual partner touch, which may in turn improve your sex life. Increased displays of nonverbal intimacy between romantic couples are generally well received and reciprocated. If you make more nonverbal intimacy gestures, it is likely that your partner will respond in kind. The exception to this rule is that if increased nonverbal cues violate expectations and are highly discrepant from expected behavior, they can cause overarousal, defensiveness, and flight. In other words, if your partner is not used to overt displays of affection and nonverbal intimacy, take it slow. Also, for a couple with normally low amounts of nonverbal intimacy, when something goes wrong, they are likely to compensate with verbal attempts. For example, if a man hugs a woman and she pulls away, he might respond verbally with "why did you pull away?" "is something wrong?" "do you still love me?" to figure out why she did not hug him back.[12]

NONVERBAL SIGNS OF SEXUAL INTEREST AND LOVE

There are many different ways to tell if someone is showing affection and is sexually interested. The most obvious nonverbal signs are affirmative head nods, Duchenne smiles (i.e., raising the cheek muscles and squinting the eyes at the corners, producing smile lines at the corner of the mouth and eyes), positive gesturing with the hands, open gestures, and leaning toward the partner. However, these are most often associated with romantic love rather than desire.[13] Nonverbal sexual cues that indicate desire revolve more around the mouth and include licking, puckering, touching the lips, tongue protrusions, biting the lips, and sucking the lips so they are rolled into the mouth.

Michael Cunningham and Anita Barbee, experts in relationship initiation, reviewed studies on nonverbal cues that attract attention of a sexual nature.[14] They believe there are four dimensions of nonverbal attraction: neonate, mature, expressive, and grooming. Neoteny explains how human beings are attracted to babyish features and cuteness. Cute, baby features include large eyes, small noses, smooth skin, shiny hair, and light coloration. Perhaps these stimuli suggest youthfulness and fitness, which are benefits of resources for mates. Despite the desirability of cuteness, Cunningham and Barbee claim that physically attractive adults possess sexually mature features. For females, this means narrow cheeks, high cheekbones, prominent breasts, long legs, and symmetrical features. For men, this means a broad chin, thick eyebrows, visible facial hair, tallness, and a deep voice. Expressive features are a part of nonverbal courting behaviors and include the expression of positive emotions and social interest through large smiles, dilated pupils, high-set eyebrows, full lips, and a confident posture. These nonverbal cues make a person appear friendly, helpful, and responsive.

The last type of nonverbal behavior is grooming. This includes hair-styles, cosmetics, body weight, possessions, and clothing. Grooming can reveal a lot about a person's sense of style, intelligence, creativity, and access to personal and social resources. For example, women can wear eye makeup to increase their expressiveness or lipstick to accentuate their lips and make them appear fuller. Men can participate in body-building to find the ideal body weight to attract women. The question of resources is yet to be researched with definitive conclusions: can a display of resources (such as an expensive car or suit) increase a person's romantic success? As far as research goes, the experts know that men use expensive cars more than women to attract attention; however, they cannot definitely conclude that this increases their sexual success.

Interestingly, another nonverbal factor that may hold just as much weight as physical attractiveness and access to resources is peer esteem; that is, those who are held in high regard by their peers, particularly those of the opposite sex, are found to be more attractive to potential partners. A variety of studies were done on both people and animals, and those who received the most attention from the opposite sex were sought out by others who observed this phenomenon. Researchers call this the *celebrity effect*.[15]

PHYSICAL PROXIMITY, INTERPERSONAL COMMUNICATION, AND SEX

Several researchers have investigated the communicative effects of physical proximity on interpersonal communication. Many communication scholars have examined how the distance people maintain from one another affects the message that is communicated about their relationship.[16] Indeed, how close people stand to one another in a social interaction has been shown to serve as an indicator of potential relational expectations.[17] Psychologist Edward Hall believes the primary purpose of physical proximity in a social interaction is to convey messages about the level of intimacy appropriate or desired for that interaction.[18] Hall has proposed that we have four distance categories for social interaction, which he calls *zones*. Within each zone, we perceive distinct cues about what level of intimacy to expect. These cues and expectations influence how we interpret relational messages sent to us by others. As people move further away from each other, the imposition of distance modifies the content of relational messages from intimate to more formal. This makes sense: the further away we are from someone, the less intimate we want the interaction to be.

The first of Hall's four zones is the *intimate zone*, a distance between people of anywhere from zero to 1-1/2 feet. This zone, which may include participant touching, maximizes sensory involvement, and intimacy is anticipated and even expected. The second zone, 1-1/2 to four feet between participants, is termed *personal distance*. This zone functions primarily as an area for conversation among friends and relatives. The third or *social zone* involves a distance between individuals of 4–10 feet. This distance is employed when greeting a visitor from a desk or when one is asking for directions from a stranger on the street. In the last or *public zone*, people are positioned 10–25 feet apart. This zone is used primarily for formal presentations, plays, speeches, and other means of public communication. At this level, sensory involvement is greatly reduced, and other objects and people compete for the person's attention. Uses of these zones are remarkably consistent within a culture. Conformity to the distance requirement of each zone may not even be noticed by most people. Most important, use of the zone or crossing from one zone to another may be considered a form of communication in itself. When a casual acquaintance engages us in an intimate zone, we may expect to hear something private. Because of this expectancy, we may come to evaluate what is being said as private in this zone, whereas exactly the same words spoken in the personal zone may convey a different message altogether.

DATING AND NONVERBAL BEHAVIOR

To interact with people, you must have some ability to convey your own level of interest and gauge the interest of the other. The more able you are to accurately do this is directly linked to your level of comfort and success in dating, relationships, and sex. There are great benefits to be able to correctly evaluate the other person's degree of interest as well as accurately convey your own level of interest. This is part of impression management—what impression you are giving your partner. One of the most difficult contexts to negotiate these communication skills, both verbal and nonverbal, is in the dating context. There is not much scientific research available that can help teach people to express verbal and nonverbal cues that accurately and appropriately convey levels of sexual interest. This is why society has celebrated non-research-based books and theories that focus on popular wisdom about dating and convey interest such as the book *He's Just Not That into You.* The popularity of such books and movies would lead us to believe that men and women are blind to verbal and nonverbal cues and that they cannot accurately assess when someone is "into them" or interested in them sexually. Perhaps that is why so much attention in our popular culture is devoted to these topics. There is little scientific research investigating these particular issues; however, there is a multitude of research that shows women have much higher rates of reading communication cues, particularly surrounding sexual intent, than do men. So then why do women spend so much time trying to evaluate if men are sexually interested in them? We can conclude that the average American is relatively lost when it comes to ascertaining if someone is romantically interested in him, particularly at the beginning of a relationship.

Coreen Ferris, a researcher at Indiana University, and her colleagues from Yale University conducted a study about sexual intent. They published their findings in an article titled "Perceptual Mechanisms That Characterize Gender Differences in Decoding Women's Sexual Intent."[19] They set out to study the level of accuracy men and women had when it came to assessing if a woman was simply being friendly or had a sexual interest in a man, particularly in early interactions. The researchers agree that "decoding sexual intent is an arguably difficult task, particularly if the perceiver hopes to decode intent early in an interaction. Women may smile, sustain eye contact, decrease physical proximity, or touch their partner to convey romantic or sexual interest. However, all of these cues also could be used to convey simple warmth, friendliness, or platonic interest." Ferris concluded that "given ambiguity in separating sexual interest from platonic interest and the overlapping nonverbal cues used to signal these two kinds of interest, it should come as no surprise that individuals often disagree about the meaning of nonverbal sexual signals."[20] This and other research has shown that men consistently rate women as intending to convey a greater degree of sexual interest than do women who rate the same targets—a finding that has been remarkably consistent across studies, ranging from those using still photographs and video vignettes to those using live, unscripted interactions.[21] Ferris provides two different theories that may explain why women are better at decoding sexual intent than men. One theory is called the *decisional-threshold* (or *bias*) *theory*, which states that men

require fewer impelling cues than women before labeling a woman's behavior as sexual.[22] According to this theory, men and women perceive
the same positive behavioral cues, but men are more likely to identify
cues as indicative of sexual interest because they have a more lenient
decisional threshold as compared to women. Conversely, women wait
for more direct sexual interest cues before being willing to apply the
label of sexual interest. Theorists have suggested that men may develop
lenient thresholds for judging sexual interest because they are socialized to be sexually zealous and dominant.

The second theory regarding the source of the gender difference
suggests that men are simply worse than women when it comes to reading all nonverbal communication cues, not just sexual cues, and that
men are less sensitive to emotional signaling in many different contexts.
So men may misinterpret sexual interest not because they have a low
threshold for labeling sexual interest, but "because they are less sensitive to women's nonverbal cues than women are and find it perceptu-
ally difficult to differentiate the subtle cues that discriminate women's
sexual interest from their platonic interest. . . . Such insensitivity may
be particularly relevant among young men who are just entering the
dating system, and therefore may not have acquired the experience necessary to reliably and accurately discriminate between women's platonic
and sexual-interest cues."[23] According to this theory, then, men are just
as likely to mistake women's sexual interest with platonic friendliness
because they are not very good at reading cues.

The research that Farris conducted supports the theory that men
are just generally worse at reading all nonverbal cues. In her research,
men were significantly worse than women at judging sexual intent. In
many cases, men tended to oversexualize some women but were quite
likely to undersexualize other women. They missed obvious cues that a
woman was sexually interested in them, as well. Overall, this study suggests that while there is a general tendency for women to be more successful than men at decoding nonverbal cues, there is a particularly
pronounced gender difference when nonverbal cues are sexual in nature.

FLIRTING

Even though some people deny that they flirt, almost everyone flirts,
single and married people alike. Flirting can be broken down into basic
nonverbal components, including gestures, eye contact, stances, and
movements. Many of these behaviors are unintentional and subtle but

are easily observed by scientists studying flirting behaviors. Research has shown that men tend to flirt because of sexual interest, while women flirt to be friendly. Highly flirtatious messages tended to be inviting, sexually assertive, overt, playful, unconventional, and nonverbal. Although men and women tend to display different messages while flirting, they tend to judge whether people are flirting with them—the intention to flirt—in similar ways. We all look out for those signals. Keep in mind that location and relationship are significant factors in determining if someone is flirting. Is the interaction taking place in a bar or in the office? Is this person your boss, brother-in-law, or single friend? Location and relationship will significantly affect the interpretation of flirtatious messages.[24]

Many evolutionary biologists claim that we cannot help but flirt; it is programmed into us, and we keep doing it even after we are married. Research has also shown that women flirt when they are nervous or unsure of themselves in a situation, even at work, because flirting behaviors are comfortable fallbacks for them; women know the rules to flirting.

Everybody has a unique way of flirting, and people interpret flirting behaviors differently. Some people are flattered when people flirt with them, some are oblivious, and some are uncomfortable. Communication professors Jeffrey Hall, Michael Cody, Grace Jackson, and Jacqueline Flesh have investigated the different styles of flirting and identified the types of communication enacted in each style.[25] They came up with six different kinds of flirting behaviors. The *physical* flirting style is used by people who flirt by expressing their physical interest in others by touching and through conversation; it is often playful flirting. Men and women use this style equally and report that they are able to discern the sexual interest of others and are willing and capable of conveying romantic interest. Often, people who prefer the physical style feel an attraction with someone quickly, move to personal and private conversation, and successfully establish the possibility of a relationship. In the most recent relationships of the respondents, those who were high on the physical flirting style reported a faster pace of relational development, with more sexual chemistry and emotional connection than those with other styles. Older age groups report more confidence in the sexual communication of romantic interest with this style. In fact, respondents aged 18–24 years scored the lowest on this style of flirting, with scores increasing as people got older, reaching a high in the 40s and then slowly declining. The physical flirting style is favored by individuals who report high levels of extraversion, openness, agreeableness, conscientiousness, and self-monitoring. Researchers concluded that people who are comfortable expressing their interest in others physically are also likely to seek an emotional connection.

Another style of flirting is called the *traditional* style because those who use this approach believe in traditional gender roles for men and women: men make the first move, and women should not pursue men. Researchers found that women who fall into this category are less likely to be able to communicate romantic attraction, are less likely to flirt with potential partners and to be flattered by flirting, and report having trouble getting men to notice their behavior. Also, women are less likely to report success with the opposite sex, feel less confident, and often fail to establish relationship potential. Traditional-flirting-style women do not immediately experience romantic attraction and are less likely to have private and personal conversations with a potential partner. The end result is decreased courtship success because women have few options to attract a mate. Even once people are in a relationship, the traditional flirting style was negatively related to experiencing sexual chemistry and emotional connection for women, but not for men. For men with high scores on the traditional style, there are also fewer mate possibilities because men report romantic interest with fewer people and are more likely to know a potential relationship partner for a longer time before approaching her. Men did not find many potential partners, and once they had identified one, they developed a nonromantic relationship before acting upon romantic desires. During the time a traditional couple is getting to know one another, a traditional woman is unlikely to be receptive to flirtation and unlikely to communicate attraction. Once a traditional woman is in a relationship, research shows she is likely to have less sexual chemistry and emotional connectedness with her partner that other kinds of flirts. The researchers speculated that if two highly traditional partners met, they would probably proceed slowly in all stages of courtship. Overall, individuals high on the traditional flirting style are younger women who are introverted and are not completely comfortable in social situations.

The *inhibited* flirt uses a guarded and rule-governed approach to flirting and relationships in general. Inhibited flirts are also more likely to use proper manners and nonsexual communication. Like those with traditional flirting styles, people report interest in fewer potential partners, and when interested, women are less likely to approach a person and less likely to finding flirting flattering. This kind of person is likely to seek out meaningful relationships and sincere connections with others, rather than flirting for superficial reasons or fun.

Most people in the research project had a *sincere* flirting style. Sincere flirts are generally extroverts, highly agreeable, conscientious of others, and open. The sincere flirt shows sincere interest and seeks an emotional connection with another person. He is willing and able to approach members of the opposite sex, to find flirting flattering, and to believe that others were flirting with him often. Through personal and private conversations with potential partners, individuals high in the sincere style report more success, more confidence, and a greater likelihood of establishing of relationship potential. Once in a relationship, the sincere flirting style was positively related to having a strong emotional connection, sexual chemistry, and an important and meaningful relationship. Sincere flirts are comfortable engaging in sexual communication.

The playful flirt builds self-esteem through flirting and often flirts for fun. The main difference in this style of flirting compared to others is that people flirt to have fun rather than establish a romantic connection; they even flirt with people with whom they have no romantic interest. When communicating with potential partners, the playful flirts report more success and self-confidence and do not establish relationship potential. This kind of flirting decreases with age. Men report the swift development of relatively unimportant relationships with higher sexual chemistry. Male and female playful flirts are generally extraverts with an outgoing nature but lack concern for other people. The researchers found that the playful flirt is able to put on a good social performance for the benefit of others. The playful flirt is likely to be comfortable expressing sexual interest and is less likely to adhere to strict politeness norms during courtship.

Nonverbal Flirting Behaviors

Communication scholars call the nonverbal signs we give off *nonverbal leakage*—those things that escape or are disclosed in a nonverbal manner—often without direct thought and intent. The signs we give off when we are flirting are nonverbal leakage and indicate that we are "contact ready." The most common signs for women are a tilt of the head, called a *head cant*, to the side to expose her neck and a Duchenne smile. Men position their bodies in an open, come-on-attack-me position, using their hands to draw attention to their lower abdomen. Both sexes display prolonged eye contact, lean into a person, and show extended attention for that person. Men who report that they are flirting smile more, laugh more, gaze downward less often, and display more frequent flirtatious glances. Women are more likely to lean forward and cant their heads.[26]

Why Do We Flirt?

In an article titled "Why Do We Flirt?" David Henningsen, Mary Braz, and Elaine Davies examine the motivations of people who engage in flirtatious behaviors in different contexts.[27] They contend, as I do, that flirting is intentionally vague for a number of reasons. They believe that flirtatious interactions intentionally promote ambiguity in terms of sexual intent behaviors. People lead a receiver to suspect that sexual interest is being expressed but with enough ambiguity that the receiver cannot confirm the presence of sexual interest. This is what flirting is, rather than directly hitting on someone. There are different goals that people have for flirting; we do not always flirt because we want to have sex with someone or begin a romantic relationship.

In recent studies,[28] Henningsen identified six motivations for flirtation. These motivations include to facilitate sexual contact (sexual motivation), to advance an existing romantic relationship (relational motivation), to have fun (fun motivation), to explore the potential for a romantic relationship (exploring motivation), to foster self-esteem (esteem motivation), and to encourage another to do something for the person (instrumental motivation). It is clear that both men and women flirt because of sexual motivation. We desire sexual contact with another person. This is directly related to how attractive we find other people. Many people report that they choose not to flirt with someone because they are not sexually attracted to them. Relational motivation means that people want to increase the intensity of a relationship. For example, behaviors identified as flirting behaviors are employed when people want to have a closer relationship with someone. In looking at the sexual and relational motivations, we can see gender differences emerge that fit with the evolutionary perspective: men are likely to pursue more sexual encounters than women, whereas women are more likely to flirt to establish relational commitment and closeness than men. Thus, generally speaking, men flirt to have sex and women flirt more to develop and intensify relationships.

The exploring motivation is when flirting is used to assess the interest another may have. People want to test how willing a person is to establish initial contact with another or how likely he or she would be to say yes if asked out on a date. Therefore it does not mean that someone is necessarily interested in the end goal of sexual contact, but would like to assess if the possibility is there and if the other person is interested. Numerous researchers from different disciplines of study, including psychology, anthropology, biology, communication, and medicine, have examined behaviors women use to increase the likelihood that men will approach them. Many popular self-help books have focused on this theme, as well. However, there is scientific research that examines ways a woman is able to gain the attention of men and get men to approach her. "This allows women to gauge different men's attraction and interest. Such behaviors, which essentially gain the attention of a cross-sex target, allow individuals to test the waters to determine the depth of interest of potential suitors. The response of the targets provides information about their attraction to the initiator. . . . Behaviors used to indicate an interest in dating logically reflect a desire to test the interest another party has in beginning a romantic relationship."[29] The researchers concluded that women consciously engage in these flirting behaviors and that men consciously respond to them.

Although individuals may flirt to promote sexual contact or relational advancement, they may also flirt simply because it is fun or because it makes them feel good about themselves. Many people flirt because it is an enjoyable and entertaining form of interaction. For instance, many individuals report that flirting can be a fun and harmless behavior.[30] It also can be used to pass the time or because it is distracting. In addition, friends engage in flirting activities even when their relationship is platonic.[31] Thus some of the benefits of flirting seem to be in the pleasure of the interaction itself, rather than in the advancement of relational or sexual goals. This may be why people often harmlessly flirt with strangers on airplane trips. It is interesting that women reported flirting for fun more than men. From an evolutionary perspective, women need to develop a large repertoire of flirting behaviors so that they are able to attract men who are good relational targets.[32] To develop such an assortment, women may need to engage in what could be called practice flirting. In essence, flirting for fun may allow women to compare effective and ineffective flirting strategies in a harmless fashion. Another researcher found that adolescent girls engaged in an array of flirting behaviors in mixed-sex situations and attributed these behaviors to refining flirting expertise.[33] Adult married women may continue to engage in practice flirting because it is enjoyable and because it promotes greater flirting skill.

People also flirt to build their own self-esteem. Some individuals feel flattered when others flirt with them.[34] If flirting behaviors are reciprocated, a person may engage in flirting to produce this effect. If people respond favorably to flirting behaviors, it may make the person who initiates flirting feel attractive, desirable, or interesting.

Last, people flirt because of instrumental motivation. In other words, they flirt with someone to gain some desired assistance or reward. A classic example is an individual in a bar who is flirting in the hope that someone will buy her a drink. Another example would be flirting with a police officer to get out of a ticket or flirting with a person in retail to get the best product or customer service. Flirting may be a useful strategy in gaining such assistance.

So, given all these reasons we flirt, why do people flirt at work? Most people at work flirt to have fun, followed by the desire to gauge whether a person is interested in them sexually (motivation), to build their self-esteem, and to get people to do things for them (instrumental).[35] Relatively few people report flirting at work due to sexual and relational motivations. Therefore people flirt in different places for different reasons. And sexual harassment issues aside, flirting at work is a relatively harmless activity used to make work more fun. Another study on flirting in the workplace found that women sometimes flirt for instrumental purposes.[36] The effectiveness of flirting in garnering instrumental rewards has been noted in the hospitality industry. A variety of hospitality outlets encourage waitstaff to flirt to increase spending and increase the repeat business of customers. Some managers considered flirting to be part of the job of service staff.[37] Likewise, have you ever met a male hair stylist that did not flirt? Even if that hair stylist is gay, it is part of the job to flirt with clients to make them feel good about themselves. This ensures good tips and repeat business.

Most people believe that flirting will get them things. For example, in a study, both male and female college students believed that flirting could help to improve their grades. In this study, sizable proportions of both men and women reported that they had flirted with their instructors.[38] Nearly three-quarters of those surveyed believed that female students could improve their grades by flirting with male faculty. One-half of the sample thought that men could raise their grades by flirting with female faculty. Although this implies that women may be better able to use flirting to accomplish their goals, it is clear that many men and women believe that flirting can get you things.

Flirting is an essential process in finding a partner, but just because a person is married does not mean he stops flirting. Flirting plays an important role between married couples, and marriage counselors encourage people to keep flirting throughout their marriage. Nonverbal communication plays an essential role in martial happiness and the quality of sex in marriages. The next section reviews some studies from interpersonal scholars about the role of nonverbal communication in marriage.

NUDITY

Nudity is a form of nonverbal communication that is directly related to sex. You could even say it is nonverbal communication about sex. How the media depict male and female nudity directly influences our own perceptions of nudity and the appropriateness of nudity. This is definitely cultural and has long been debated in the international press. For example, there are more depictions of gratuitous sex and nudity in American movies than in any other countries, yet as a culture, Americans are very uncomfortable with nudity in person or public. Some beaches in Florida recently banned thong bikinis, yet in many European countries, people sunbath topless without shame. Appropriate displays of nudity are obviously culturally determined; there is compelling evidence that how we view nudity is culturally influenced and even influenced by gender. Research shows that men and women have different reactions to nudity. First, there is a large quantity of evidence substantiating a rather obvious truism: men are interested in and sexually aroused by the sight of a nude woman.[39]

Some research has shown that women are less aroused by the sight of male nudity. When college men viewed nude female photos in *Playboy* and women viewed nude male photos in *Playgirl*, the men and women reported different degrees of sexual interest and arousal. The results showed that 88 percent of men rated the nude female photos as "sexually interesting," but only 46 percent of women rated the nude male photos as such.[40] Furthermore, when the people reported their degree of sexual stimulation in response to the photos, 75 percent of men reported being highly stimulated. In addition to sexual interest and arousal, men exposed to nude females experienced a change in their emotional state and showed changes in attitudes toward objects associated with female nudity. Research on consumer reactions to nudity in advertisements suggests that men, compared to women, show more positive emotional arousal and positive attitudes toward a product after viewing ads for the product containing female nudity.[41]

Changes in emotional reactions among males have also been found to occur in response to female nudity in other contexts. Other researchers found that subjects who saw nude photographs reported feeling less bored and more pleased than when viewing other stimuli.[42] In another study, men exposed to nude females were also less likely to exhibit aggressive behavior toward a female confederate of the experimenter immediately after viewing the nudes. This finding, that men are less likely to be aggressive after seeing nudity, appears to be robust.[43] In yet another study, researchers exposed men to either neutral control stimuli (such as a photo of a dog) or pictures of nude females in an investigation of the effects of erotic stimuli on subsequent aggression.[44] Exposure to nudity inhibited men's aggression toward females they were later asked to punish. Those who saw the neutral photos showed no reduction in aggression. Researchers have even tested men's reactions to nude and semiclad women.[45] Men who were shown nude photographs of women showed lower levels of aggression toward a female compared to men who viewed semiclad women and the neutral photographs. In combination, these behavioral studies of aggression suggest that when males are exposed to nude females, they experience effects that are noticeably different than reactions to semiclad females or neutral stimuli. The explanations for these findings vary according to each research group. Perhaps the most compelling is offered by Baron, who conducted the study between semiclothed and naked women: he suggests that the erotic messages conveyed by the nude female stimuli induce a state of mind that appears to be incompatible with aggressive thoughts and behaviors.

NONVERBAL COMMUNICATION AND MARRIAGE

In a study of nonverbal communication and martial happiness, Ascan F. Koerner and Mary Anne Fitzpatrick found that nonverbal communication is directly related to marital happiness.[46] Basically, couples who accurately decode and encode nonverbal messages are happier in their marriages. If a wife can accurately read her husband's nonverbal messages and in turn send out nonverbal messages that he can accurately understand, then this couple may have an easier adjustment to marriage and overall higher rates of martial happiness. Other research has shown that this largely depends on the man's communication skills because women, on the whole, are good at encoding and decoding nonverbal messages, whereas men generally have a much harder time. So it is safe to say that if the man in the relationship is good at nonverbal communication, then it is a happier marriage. Much of what we communicate about the state of our relationships is done nonverbally rather than in the content of our verbal messages, especially in marital relationships. Koerner and Fitzpatrick theorize that a spouse's ability to differentiate whether the affect (experience of feeling or emotion) that her partner communicates is caused by the relationship or is caused by factors external to the relationship is very important for relationship success.

For example, in many conversations, people get a feeling that their spouses are unhappy or not willing to talk, but those who have happy marriages are able to tell when a spouse is in a certain mood due to the relationship or due to something else, perhaps a problem at work or a fight with a friend. Therefore one essential skill spouses need to work on is decoding whether the nonverbal affect in a message reflects the sender's feelings about the relationship or partner (relational), or whether the nonverbal affect reflects factors unrelated to the relationship or partner (nonrelational). Sometimes partners will be able to make accurate relational or nonrelational attributions based on contextual cues or based on verbal message content. In situations where these cues are ambiguous, however, partners have to rely on decoding the nonverbal behaviors of their spouses. In other words, if a husband is able to recognize if his wife is unhappy with him or is really unhappy about something external to the relationship, then it is much better for the relationship. It is of equal importance that when assessing and negotiating relationships, spouses are able to successfully communicate their affects regarding the relationship. It takes skill in both accurately sending messages and decoding messages. Thus, for spouses to understand their partners and to negotiate their relationships successfully, they must pay attention to subtle emotional cues within nonverbal communication.

So what are the nonverbal signs (the nonverbal leakage) that you can look for to help you determine if a person is happy because of the relationship or something external to the relationship? Likewise, what are the cues to help you understand if a person is upset with something in the relationship (or you) or something external to the relationship? There are nonverbal signs or cues that are related to positive interpersonal interaction. These are often experienced in the form of love and affection, which are closely associated with fondness, liking, attraction, and longing. Nonverbal manifestations of affection include prolonged eye contact, closer interpersonal distance, blushing, pupil dilation, increased smiling, and increased and prolonged touch across many areas of the body.[47] Nonrelational positive affect is often experienced in the form of pleasure. Pleasure is often associated with happiness, one of the basic human emotions. Pleasure is represented nonverbally by the

Duchenne smile; increased vocal pitch, intensity, and rate; a melodious tone of voice; and more laughing, touching, and close interpersonal distances.[48]

In general, negative feelings about the relationship are often experienced in the form of anger and irritation, while negative feelings about things external to the relationship are exhibited with signs of sadness. Anger, also considered one of the basic emotions, involves an intense feeling of displeasure that results from being injured, harmed, or mistreated. It is usually the result of interpersonal interaction, although it also can occur outside of interpersonal relationships. Anger has a characteristic facial expression: a direct stare, knit and lowered brows, narrowed eyes, and a tense jaw with the mouth often open and the teeth exposed. The angry voice is louder, harsher, and deeper in pitch.[49] When something is bothering someone that is external to the marriage, it usually shows up in feelings of sadness and depression. Sadness and depression are characterized by a chronic sad affect, melancholy feelings, and a host of other symptoms. The facial presentation of sadness is easily recognized with a downturned mouth and downturned eyes. Behavioral signs of sadness include a slumping posture, frowning, moping, a lowered head, prolonged silences, withdrawal, social isolation, talking in a monotone, lowered vocal volume, decreased smiling, reduced eye contact, and in extreme cases, crying and sobbing.[50] So it will definitely help you to recognize when your spouse is upset due to something in the relationship or outside of the relationship. Look for these cues.

IMPROVING YOUR NONVERBAL COMMUNICATION SKILLS

In this chapter, the role of nonverbal communication in sexual relationships was reviewed. Nonverbal communication is important to establish and enhance sexual and romantic relationships. We use nonverbal cues to let people know if we want to have sex with them and what we like during sex. The ability to accurately assess nonverbal cues is of great importance, and it has been shown that in general, women are better at it than men. There are many ways to improve your nonverbal communication skills. First, I review the different kinds of problematic communication so you know how to better improve certain skills.

In a book titled *The Nonverbal Communication Reader: Classic and Contemporary Readings*, authors Michael Hecht, Joseph DeVito, and Laura Guerrero described three forms of imperfect communication: miscommunication, attempted communication, and misinterpretation.[51] *Mis-*

communication reflects instances where the meaning attributed to an intentional message by the receiver is different than that intended by the sender. In the context of sex, we can look at the example of gender differences in the perceptions of women's sexual interest. A miscommunication would occur if a woman engaged in behavior with a nonsexual intent that was interpreted as sexual by a man. This happens frequently, but men never stop to say, "Hey, were you flirting with me?" or "Are you interested in a sexual relationship with me?"; rather, they just assume that a woman was interested. It would be very awkward if these kinds of questions were asked, and chances are a woman would not be honest. This is a form of miscommunication.

Attempted communication is a process by which a sender conveys a message that is not received by the receiver. For example, if, during a cross-sex interaction, a woman intentionally sends a message indicating a lack of sexual interest in her male counterpart that the man does not perceive, attempted communication could lead to gender differences in perceptions of sexual interest. A woman may try to send a direct signal that she is not interested: she may physically pull back and end eye contact or send a verbal message such as "my boyfriend is waiting for me," but surprisingly, often men do not pick up on these cues. Finally, if a sender unintentionally sends a message that a receiver interprets as conveying a specific intent, *misinterpretation* occurs. Thus, if a man interprets a woman's wink as an indicator of sexual interest when, in fact, the woman merely displayed an involuntary twitch, misinterpretation would lead to imperfect communication of sexual interest.

It is unclear whether understanding body movements and paralinguistic cues can help you improve nonverbal communication skills because so much of nonverbal communication is spontaneous. However, most experts agree that with work, people can improve their skills if they try. For example, you can try to anticipate reactions you might have if you initiate a discussion about sex and practice maintaining eye contact when you are discussing this topic. Be prepared for unexpected answers, surprises, or perhaps even disappointment. One reason that people are so reluctant to talk about sex and, in particular, their own sexual experiences with their partners is because they are afraid that they may hurt someone's feelings. It is tough to be criticized in general, particularly about something as intimate as sex. By talking about sex, we may be inviting criticism about our performances or our partners' performances, and we have to be ready for that. Most people are reluctant to open this Pandora's box for numerous reasons. Perhaps previous attempts in the past have not been received well, or there is a fear of hurting our partner's feelings or fear that our partner may not want sex anymore if he or she feels bad about his or her performance. Some people feel that mediocre or infrequent sex is better than no sex at all, and it is not worth the risk to talk about it to try to make it better. Some people may start a conversation and not even give the other person time to respond because of the look on the other person's face. They might say something like, "Oh, I know I should not have even brought this up, I can tell by the look on your face that you are upset. I am sorry. Forget I ever said anything. Really, things are fine the way they are."

One way to counteract nonverbal cues is to say something like "please do not think that I don't want to hear what you are saying. The fact is that I do want to hear it, but I automatically frown when I am criticized. I cannot help this, but I really want to talk about this issue" or "I know sex is a serious topic, but I cannot help but smile or giggle when we talk about it, please, this is just a nervous reaction I cannot help. Please continue." Many people have practice sex talks in their head, aloud, or with friends before they try it out on the real person. This is particularly common between parents and sexually mature adolescents. People practice their main messages, anticipate questions and responses, and try to increase their persuasiveness. During this time, try to practice your nonverbal cues, as well. Maintain a calm voice (paralinguistic cues), maintain eye contact, and do not physically withdraw from the conversation. This will help you regulate your nonverbal cues.

Do not be afraid to check your nonverbal perceptions. If you think you are reading a cue correctly, ask the other person about it. "Oh, I see from the smile on your face that you think this funny. Am I off base?" You may be surprised at the response—you never know why a person is smiling; it may also be that the person is embarrassed and trying to save face or that the person had a feeling you wanted to talk about sex and was smiling because the person was right. By asking the person directly how she is feeling, you can have more meaningful conversations and less miscommunications that might shut down a conversation.

NOTES

1. Carey M. Noland, "Listening to the Sound of Silence: Gender Roles and Communication about Sex in Puerto Rico," *Sex Roles* 55, no. 5 (2006).

2. Mark Knapp and Judith Hall, *Nonverbal Communication in Human Interaction*, 5th ed. (Belmont CA: Wadsworth/Thomson Learning, 2002), 350.

3. Julia Wood, *Gendered Lives*, 7th ed. (Belmont, CA: Thompson Wadsworth, 2007), 138.

4. Irvin Goffman, *Interaction Rituals: Essays on Face to Face Behavior* (Garden City, NY: Doubleday, 1967). Judee Burgoon, Joseph Walther, and James Baesler, "Interpretations, Evaluations, and Consequences of Interpersonal Touch," *Human Communication Research* 19, no. 2 (1992).

5. Stanley E. Jones and Elaine Yarbrough, "A Naturalistic Study of the Meanings of Touch," *Communication Monographs* 52, no. 1 (1985).

6. Ibid.

7. Laura K. Guerrero and Peter A. Andersen, "The Waxing and Waning of Relational Intimacy: Touch as a Function of Relational Stage, Gender and Touch Avoidance," *Journal of Social and Personal Relationships* 8, no. 2 (1991).

8. Fredric E. Rabinowitz, "The Male-to-Male Embrace: Breaking the Touch Taboo in a Men's Therapy Group," *Journal of Counseling and Development* 69, no. 6 (1991).

9. Guerrero and Andersen, "Waxing and Waning."

10. Richard Heslin, Tuan D. Nguyen, and Michele L. Nguyen, "Meaning of Touch: The Case of Touch from a Stranger or Same Sex Person," *Journal of Nonverbal Behavior* 7, no. 3 (1983).

11. Nicolas Gueguen and Jacques Fischer-Lokou, "Another Evaluation of Touch and Helping Behavior," *Psychological Reports* 92, no. 1 (2003).

12. Laura K. Guerrero, Susanne M. Jones, and Judee K. Burgoon, "Responses to Nonverbal Intimacy Change in Romantic Dyads: Effects of Behavioral Valence and Degree of Behavioral Change on Nonverbal and Verbal Reactions," *Communication Monograph* 67, no. 4 (2000).

13. Gian Gonzaga, Dacher Keltner, Esme Londahl, and Michael Smith, "Love and the Commitment Problem in Romantic Relations and Friendship," *Journal of Personality and Social Psychology* 81, no. 2 (2001).

14. Michael Cunningham and Anita Barbee, "Prelude to a Kiss: Nonverbal Flirting, Opening Gambits, and Other Communication Dynamics in the Initiation of Romantic Relationships," in *Handbook of Relationship Initiation*, ed. Susan Sprecher, Amy Wenzel, and John Harvey (New York: Psychology Press, 2008).

15. Ibid.

16. Judee Burgoon, "Nonverbal Violations of Expectations," in *Nonverbal Interaction*, ed. J.M. Wiemann and R.P. Harrison (Beverly Hills, CA: Sage, 1983).

17. Beth A. Le Poire and Judee K. Burgoon, "Two Contrasting Explanations of Involvement Violations: Expectancy Violations Theory versus Discrepancy Arousal Theory," *Human Communication Research* 20 (1994).

18. Edward Hall, *The Silent Language* (Garden City, NY: Anchor Press, 1973).

19. Coreen Farris, Teresa A. Treat, Richard J. Viken, and Richard M. McFall, "Perceptual Mechanisms That Characterize Gender Differences in Decoding Women's Sexual Intent," *Psychological Science* 19 (2008).

20. Ibid., 348.

21. Antonia Abbey, "Misperceptions of Friendly Behavior as Sexual Interest: A Survey of Naturally Occurring Incidents," *Psychology of Women Quarterly* 11, no. 2 (1987). R. Lance Shotland and Jane M. Craig, "Can Men and Women Differentiate between Friendly and Sexually Interested Behavior?" *Social Psychology Quarterly* 51, no. 1 (1988).

22. Martie G. Haselton and Daniel Nettle, "The Paranoid Optimist: An Integrative Evolutionary Model of Cognitive Biases," *Personality and Social Psychology Review* 10, no. 1 (2006).

23. Farris et al., "Perceptual Mechanisms."

24. Matthew F. Abrahams, "Perceiving Flirtatious Communication: An Exploration of the Perceptual Dimensions Underlying Judgments of Flirtatiousness," *Journal of Sex Research* 31 (1994).

25. Jeffrey Hall, Michael Cody, Grace Jackson, and Jacqueline Flesh, "Beauty and the Flirt: Attractiveness and Approaches to Relationship Initiation," In *International Communication Association*, 1–14. Montreal, Canada: International Communication Association, 2008.

26. Jeffry A. Simpson, Steven W. Gangestad, and Michael Biek, "Personality and Nonverbal Social Behavior: An Ethological Perspective of Relationship Initiation," *Journal of Experimental Social Psychology* 29, no. 5 (1993).

27. David Dryden Henningsen, Mary Braz, and Elaine Davies, "Why Do We Flirt?" *Journal of Business Communication* 45 (2008).

28. David Dryden Henningsen, "Flirting with Meaning: An Examination of Miscommunication in Flirting Interactions," *Sex Roles* 50, no. 7 (2004). David Dryden Henningsen, Mary Lynn Miller Henningsen, and Kathleen S. Valde, "Gender Differences in Perceptions of Women's Sexual Interest during Cross-Sex Interactions: An Application and Extension of Cognitive Valence Theory," *Sex Roles* 54, no. 11 (2006).

29. Henningsen, "Flirting with Meaning," 483.

30. Liana Koeppel, Yvette Montagne-Miller, Dan O'Hair, and Michael Cody, " Friendly? Flirting? Wrong?" in *Interpersonal Communication: Evolving Interpersonal Relationships*, ed. Pamela Kalbfleisch (Hillsdale, NJ: Lawrence Erlbaum Associates, 1993).

31. Kori I. Egland, Brian H. Spitzberg, and Michelle M. Zormeier, "Flirtation and Conversational Competence in Cross-Sex Platonic and Romantic Relationships," *Communication Reports* 9 (1996).

32. Melanie Trost and Jess Alberts, "An Evolutionary View on Understanding Sex Effects in Communicating Attraction," in *Sex Differences and Similarities in Communication: Critical Essays and Empirical Investigations of Sex and Gender in Interaction*, ed. Daniel Canary and Kathryn Dindia (Mahwah, NJ: Lawrence Erlbaum Associates, 1998).

33. Monica Moore, "Courtship Signaling and Adolescents: 'Girls Just Wanna Have Fun'?" *Journal of Sex Research* 32, no. 4 (1995).

34. Jerrold L. Downey and William F. Vitulli, "Self-Report Measures of Behavioral Attributions Related to Interpersonal Flirtation Situations," *Psychological Reports* 61, no. 3 (1987).

35. Henningsen et al., "Why Do We Flirt?"

36. Kevin Yelvington, "Flirting in the Factory," *Journal of the Royal Anthropological Institute* 2 (1996).

37. Yvonne Guerrier and Jonathan Guy David Gilbert, "Sexual Harassment Issues in the Hospitality Industry," *International Journal of Contemporary Hospitality Management* 10 (1998).

38. David Rowland, Larry Crisler, and Donna Cox, "Flirting between College Students and Faculty," *Journal of Sex Research* 18, no. 4 (1982).

39. Alfred Kinsey, Wardell Pomeroy, and Clyde Martin, *Sexual Behavior in the Human Male* (Philadelphia: W.B. Saunders, 1948). Alfred C. Kinsey, Wardell B. Pomeroy, Clyde E. Martin, and Paul H. Gebhard, *Sexual Behavior in the Human Female* (Oxford: Saunders, 1953).

40. John Stauffer and Richard Frost, "Male and Female Interest in Sexually-Oriented Magazines," *Journal of Communication* 26 (1976).

41. Ben B. Judd Jr. and M. Wayne Alexander, "On the Reduced Effectiveness of Some Sexually Suggestive Ads," *Journal of the Academy of Marketing Science* 11, no. 2 (1983).

42. D. Zillmann and B.S. Sapolsky, "What Mediates the Effect of Mild Erotica on Annoyance and Hostile Behavior in Males?" *Journal of Personality and Social Psychology* 35, no. 8 (1977).

43. Ibid.

44. E. Donnerstein, M. Donnerstein, and R. Evans, "Erotic Stimuli and Aggression: Facilitation or Inhibition," *Journal of Personality and Social Psychology* 32, no. 2 (1975).

45. Robert A. Baron, "Sexual Arousal and Physical Aggression: The Inhibiting Influence of 'Cheesecake' and Nudes," *Bulletin of the Psychonomic Society* 3, no. 5 (1974).

46. Ascan F. Koerner and Mary Anne Fitzpatrick, "Nonverbal Communication and Marital Adjustment and Satisfaction: The Role of Decoding Relationship Relevant and Relationship Irrelevant Affect," *Communication Monographs* 69, no. 1 (2002).

47. Peter Andersen, *Nonverbal Communication: Forms and Function* (Mountain View, CA: Mayfield, 1999).

48. Ibid., 36.

49. Daniel J. Canary, Brian H. Spitzberg, Beth A. Semic, Peter A. Andersen, and Laura K. Guerrero, "The Experience and Expression of Anger in Interpersonal Settings," in *Handbook of Communication and Emotion: Research, Theory, Applications, and Contexts* (San Diego, CA: Academic Press, 1998).

50. Chris Segrin and Mary Anne Fitzpatrick, "Depression and Verbal Aggressiveness in Different Marital Types," *Communication Studies* 43 (1992).

51. Michael Hecht, Joseph DeVito, and Laura Guerrero, "Perspectives on Nonverbal Communication: Codes, Functions, and Contexts," in *The Nonverbal Communication Reader: Classic and Contemporary Readings*, ed. Laura Guerrero, Jospeh DeVito, and Micahel Hecht (Prospect Heights, IL: Waveland Press, 1999).

REFERENCES

Abbey, Antonia. "Misperceptions of Friendly Behavior as Sexual Interest: A Survey of Naturally Occurring Incidents." *Psychology of Women Quarterly* 11, no. 2 (1987): 173–94.

Abrahams, Matthew F. "Perceiving Flirtatious Communication: An Exploration of the Perceptual Dimensions Underlying Judgments of Flirtatiousness." *Journal of Sex Research* 31 (1994): 283–92.

Andersen, Peter. *Nonverbal Communication: Forms and Function.* Mountain View, CA: Mayfield, 1999.

Baron, Robert A. "Sexual Arousal and Physical Aggression: The Inhibiting Influence of 'Cheesecake' and Nudes." *Bulletin of the Psychonomic Society* 3, no. 5 (1974): 337–39.

Burgoon, Judee. "Nonverbal Violations of Expectations." In *Nonverbal Interaction*, edited by J. M. Wiemann and R. P. Harrison, 77–111. Beverly Hills, CA: Sage, 1983.

Burgoon, Judee, Joseph Walther, and James Baesler. "Interpretations, Evaluations, and Consequences of Interpersonal Touch." *Human Communication Research* 19, no. 2 (1992): 237–63.

Canary, Daniel J., Brian H. Spitzberg, Beth A. Semic, Peter A. Andersen, and Laura K. Guerrero. "The Experience and Expression of Anger in Interpersonal Settings." In *Handbook of Communication and Emotion: Research, Theory, Applications, and Contexts*, 189–213. San Diego, CA: Academic Press, 1998.

Cunningham, Michael, and Anita Barbee. "Prelude to a Kiss: Nonverbal Flirting, Opening Gambits, and Other Communication Dynamics in the Initiation of Romantic Relationships." In *Handbook of Relationship Initiation*, edited by Susan Sprecher, Amy Wenzel, and John Harvey, 97–120. New York: Psychology Press, 2008.

Donnerstein, E., M. Donnerstein, and R. Evans. "Erotic Stimuli and Aggression: Facilitation or Inhibition." *Journal of Personality and Social Psychology* 32, no. 2 (1975): 237–44.

Downey, Jerrold L., and William F. Vitulli. "Self-Report Measures of Behavioral Attributions Related to Interpersonal Flirtation Situations." *Psychological Reports* 61, no. 3 (1987): 899–904.

Egland, Kori I., Brian H. Spitzberg, and Michelle M. Zormeier. "Flirtation and Conversational Competence in Cross-Sex Platonic and Romantic Relationships." *Communication Reports* 9 (1996): 105–17.

Farris, Coreen, Teresa A. Treat, Richard J. Viken, and Richard M. McFall. "Perceptual Mechanisms That Characterize Gender Differences in Decoding Women's Sexual Intent." *Psychological Science* 19 (2008): 348–54.

Gilbert, David, Yvonne Guerrier, and Jonathan Guy. "Sexual Harassment Issues in the Hospitality Industry." *International Journal of Contemporary Hospitality Management* 10 (1998): 48–53.

Goffman, Irvin. *Interaction Rituals: Essays on Face to Face Behavior.* Garden City, NY: Doubleday, 1967.

Gonzaga, Gian, Dacher Keltner, Esme Londahl, and Michael Smith. "Love and the Commitment Problem in Romantic Relations and Friendship." *Journal of Personality and Social Psychology* 81, no. 2 (2001): 247–62.

Gueguen, Nicolas, and Jacques Fischer-Lokou. "Another Evaluation of Touch and Helping Behavior." *Psychological Reports* 92, no. 1 (2003): 62–64.

Guerrero, Laura K., and Peter A. Andersen. "The Waxing and Waning of Relational Intimacy: Touch as a Function of Relational Stage, Gender and Touch Avoidance." *Journal of Social and Personal Relationships* 8, no. 2 (1991): 147–65.

Guerrero, Laura K., Susanne M. Jones, and Judee K. Burgoon. "Responses to Nonverbal Intimacy Change in Romantic Dyads: Effects of Behavioral Valence and Degree of Behavioral Change on Nonverbal and Verbal Reactions." *Communication Monograph* 67, no. 4 (2000): 325–46.

Hall, Edward. *The Silent Language.* Garden City, NY: Anchor Press, 1973.

Haselton, Martie G., and Daniel Nettle. "The Paranoid Optimist: An Integrative Evolutionary Model of Cognitive Biases." *Personality and Social Psychology Review* 10, no. 1 (2006): 47–66.

Hecht, Michael, Joseph DeVito, and Laura Guerrero. "Perspectives on Nonverbal Communication: Codes, Functions, and Contexts." In *The Nonverbal Communication Reader: Classic and Contemporary Readings*, edited by Laura Guerrero, Joseph DeVito, and Michael Hecht, 3–18. Prospect Heights, IL: Waveland Press, 1999.

Henningsen, David Dryden. "Flirting with Meaning: An Examination of Miscommunication in Flirting Interactions." *Sex Roles* 50, no. 7 (2004): 481–89.

Henningsen, David Dryden, Mary Braz, and Elaine Davies. "Why Do We Flirt?" *Journal of Business Communication* 45 (2008): 483–502.

Henningsen, David Dryden, Mary Lynn Miller Henningsen, and Kathleen S. Valde. "Gender Differences in Perceptions of Women's Sexual Interest during Cross-Sex Interactions: An Application and Extension of Cognitive Valence Theory." *Sex Roles* 54, no. 11 (2006): 821–29.

Heslin, Richard, Tuan D. Nguyen, and Michele L. Nguyen. "Meaning of Touch: The Case of Touch from a Stranger or Same Sex Person." *Journal of Nonverbal Behavior* 7, no. 3 (1983): 147–57.

Jones, Stanley E., and Elaine Yarbrough. "A Naturalistic Study of the Meanings of Touch." *Communication Monographs* 52, no. 1 (1985): 19–56.

Judd, Ben B., Jr., and M. Wayne Alexander. "On the Reduced Effectiveness of Some Sexually Suggestive Ads." *Journal of the Academy of Marketing Science* 11, no. 2 (1983): 156–69.

Kinsey, Alfred C., Wardell B. Pomeroy, Clyde E. Martin, and Paul H. Gebhard. *Sexual Behavior in the Human Female.* Oxford: Saunders, 1953.

Kinsey, Alfred, Wardell Pomeroy, and Clyde Martin. *Sexual Behavior in the Human Male.* Philadelphia: W. B. Saunders, 1948.

Knapp, Mark, and Judith Hall. *Nonverbal Communication in Human Interaction.* 5th ed. Belmont, CA: Wadsworth/Thomson Learning, 2002.

Koeppel, Liana, Yvette Montagne-Miller, Dan O'Hair, and Michael Cody. "Friendly? Flirting? Wrong?" In *Interpersonal Communication: Evolving Interpersonal Relationships,* edited by Pamela Kalbfleisch, 13–32. Hillsdale, NJ: Lawrence Erlbaum Associates, 1993.

Koerner, Ascan F., and Mary Anne Fitzpatrick. "Nonverbal Communication and Marital Adjustment and Satisfaction: The Role of Decoding Relationship Relevant and Relationship Irrelevant Affect." *Communication Monographs* 69, no. 1 (2002): 33–52.

Le Poire, Beth A., and Judee K. Burgoon. "Two Contrasting Explanations of Involvement Violations: Expectancy Violations Theory versus Discrepancy Arousal Theory." *Human Communication Research* 20 (1994): 560–91.

Moore, Monica. "Courtship Signaling and Adolescents: 'Girls Just Wanna Have Fun'?" *Journal of Sex Research* 32, no. 4 (1995): 319–28.

Noland, Carey M. "Listening to the Sound of Silence: Gender Roles and Communication about Sex in Puerto Rico." *Sex Roles* 55, no. 5 (2006): 283–94.

Rabinowitz, Fredric E. "The Male-to-Male Embrace: Breaking the Touch Taboo in a Men's Therapy Group." *Journal of Counseling and Development* 69, no. 6 (1991): 574–76.

Rowland, David, Larry Crisler, and Donna Cox. "Flirting between College Students and Faculty." *Journal of Sex Research* 18, no. 4 (1982): 346–59.

Segrin, Chris, and Mary Anne Fitzpatrick. "Depression and Verbal Aggressiveness in Different Marital Types." *Communication Studies* 43 (1992): 79–91.

Shotland, R. Lance, and Jane M. Craig. "Can Men and Women Differentiate between Friendly and Sexually Interested Behavior?" *Social Psychology Quarterly* 51, no. 1 (1988): 66–73.

Simpson, Jeffry A., Steven W. Gangestad, and Michael Biek. "Personality and Nonverbal Social Behavior: An Ethological Perspective of Relationship Initiation." *Journal of Experimental Social Psychology* 29, no. 5 (1993): 434–61.

Stauffer, John, and Richard Frost. "Male and Female Interest in Sexually-Oriented Magazines." *Journal of Communication* 26 (1976): 25–30.

Trost, Melanie, and Jess Alberts. "An Evolutionary View on Understanding Sex Effects in Communicating Attraction." In *Sex Differences and Similarities in Communication: Critical Essays and Empirical Investigations of Sex and Gender in Interaction,* edited by Daniel Canary and Kathryn Dindia, 233–55. Mahwah, NJ: Lawrence Erlbaum Associates, 1998.

Wood, Julia. *Gendered Lives.* 7th ed. Belmont, CA: Thompson Wadsworth, 2007.

Yelvington, Kevin. "Flirting in the Factory." *Journal of the Royal Anthropological Institute* 2 (1996): 313–33.

Zillmann, D., and B. S. Sapolsky. "What Mediates the Effect of Mild Erotica on Annoyance and Hostile Behavior in Males?" *Journal of Personality and Social Psychology* 35, no. 8 (1977): 587–96.

CHAPTER 5

Casual Sex, Friends with Benefits, and Hooking Up

Jeff and Henry played soccer together in high school and have been friends ever since. They went to the same college and now work in the same city. For the most part, they hang out with the same group of friends, with the exception of a few people from work. They are both friends with a woman named Liz, who came to their group a few years ago. Liz and Jeff have strong sexual chemistry and were thinking about starting a friends-with-benefits relationship.

"So, you think we should become friends with benefits?" Jeff asked Liz one day.

"Well, I don't see why not. We are both single now and could be great together sexually. We both want the same thing, right?" Liz replied.

"Yeah, sure, we both want to be able to hook up without having to deal with all the relationship and dating crap. We do not want to have to deal with dirty, potentially diseased strangers or wait until we are drunk to make it acceptable to do it."

Liz thought about what he said for a minute. "So, from what you said, you want to be able to hook up with me, not wait until we are drunk. What about everyone else? Should we keep this a secret? Aren't you best friends with Henry and tell him everything?"

Jeff was quick to answer her. "Yes, I am sure we should keep this secret. We don't want anyone to find out because it might mess up the dynamic of the group. Plus, what we do is our business, nobody else needs to know. I know you because we have been friends for a while; you never kiss and tell anyway."

"Yeah, somehow it feels like lying, though. And you know Amy, she is always trying to set me up. I mean, I guess I should keep going out with her setups, right? Are you OK with that?"

"Yeah, I think we should make some ground rules if we are going to become friends with benefits. After all, we are first and foremost friends. I think you should continue to date people, I don't want to hold you up or anything. I want you to be happy and I care about you. Most of all, I don't want either of us to get hurt, so we have to promise no falling in love or getting hurt. OK?"

"I agree completely. No getting hurt for either one of us. And we keep this thing a secret. Our own little secret. Now, I will see you next week sometime, right?"

INTRODUCTION

The way men and women relate to one another sexually has changed dramatically over the last few decades. The amount of news media dedicated to the evolving sexual networks of young people has been steadily increasing over the last decade. From newspaper headlines about elementary school children involved in sex parties to the proliferation of oral sex among adolescents to the college students who hook up, one thing is certain: past conceptions and ideas regarding dating and monogamous relationships are evolving and changing. While most people can identify traditional dating scripts, they no longer apply to most of today's heterosexual adolescents and people in their 20s. Many people believe that the majority of single people today do not date in a traditional sense, and in turn, this has affected how we relate to others and communicate about sex with our sexual partners, friends, family, and medical providers alike. While many authors and researchers claim that casual sex is limited to emerging and young adults, it is a more universal phenomenon among single older adults than many think. Casual sex, friends with benefits, and hooking up have become part of the American sexual landscape. The media certainly endorse nontraditional sexual practices, as well, making them seem more normal than outrageous, deviant behaviors.

There have been numerous books and articles published in the last few years that lament the death of dating and the birth of casual sex and hooking up. Rather than debating the costs and benefits of casual sex, I approach it as "it is what it is" and work within the current sexual paradigm for many people. In some ways, casual sex is liberating for many people. The bottom line is that we are in a new age of sexuality, with Internet dating, hooking up, and friends with benefits.

What makes someone willing to invite a stranger back to her apartment or accept an invitation to have sex after a few dates? People differ in their willingness to enter into casual sexual situations. Researchers Edward Herold, Eleanor Maticka-Tyndale, and Dawn Mewhinney set out to answer this question.[1] They also wanted to explain the formation of intentions to engage in casual sex. What is the likelihood that a person would, when he was out to have a good time, have sex with someone he had just met? They found that the strongest influences on intentions to engage in casual sex were personal standards, situational expectations, and previous casual sex experience. Also, peer endorsement of casual sex was significant for men. Researchers believe that behavior in any situation is a function partly of intentions, partly of habitual responses, and partly of situational constraints and conditions. Therefore, if people want to go out and hook up, they intend to hook up, and so this significantly increases the likelihood that they will have casual sex. Intention is influenced by social and affective factors as well as by rational deliberations. Social factors are the personal norms, roles, and self-concepts that belong to each person. Specifically, norms are the social rules about what should and should not be done. Is it unacceptable to have casual sex? Acceptable? Or even encouraged? *Personal roles* are behaviors that are considered appropriate for persons holding particular positions in a group, whereas *self-concept* refers to the idea that a person has of himself, the goals that it is appropriate for the person to seek or avoid, and the behaviors that the person does or does not actually engage in. Therefore that men are significantly influenced to hook up by their peer groups would account for the increased intention that many men have to engage in casual sex. According to these researchers, the decision to hook up is therefore influenced by a number of factors. The likelihood of a person to hook up can be answered by a series of questions: is it normal or encouraged by the peer group? Does a person believe it is appropriate to hook up? Does the person perceive limited negative consequences to hooking up? If the answer to these questions is yes, then it significantly increases the likelihood a person will hook up.

Many other factors play a role in an individual's decision to hook up. Factors such as shyness, fear of rejection, and simply a lack of interest in casual sex are important. According to Michael Cunningham and Anita Barbee, experts on relationship initiation, differences in preferences for short-term sexual encounters greatly affect communication during relationship initiation.[2] People who desire short-term relationships and demonstrate enthusiasm for one-night stands, numerous sexual partners, and participation in uncommitted sexual relationships are called *unrestricted* people by researchers. Interestingly, unrestricted behaviors have been found to be stable across cultures; however, it was found that certain cultural circumstances did lead to more unrestricted behaviors. These include societies where males are in short supply; women have more economic, political, and relational power; and there is a tendency toward more unrestrictive behaviors. On the flip side, societies in which women are in short supply; in which women have little economic, political, and relational power; and where the ecology is more stressful have much less unrestrictive sexual attitudes. In the United States, unrestricted sexual behaviors have taken the form of hookups and friends with benefits.

HOOKING UP

Hooking up is a distinctive sex-without-commitment interaction that is widespread in the United States. It is particularly common on college campuses and profoundly influences sexual culture on campuses. The term *hooking up* is ambiguous and could mean any sexual act ranging from kissing to sex. Hooking up can be characterized by physical intimacy rather than emotional intimacy between two people. People hook up with friends, acquaintances, and sometimes strangers. Hooking up comes from the 1960s and 1970s free-love movement, when causal sex became more mainstream. In the 1980s and 1990s, the hookup was known as a one-night stand; however, a one-night stand implies sexual intercourse, whereas a hookup could mean a variety of sexual behaviors. It could be more widespread today because of the availability of protection (condoms), increased numbers of friendships between men and women, and the fact that many young people delay marriage until later in life.

Studies have found that around 85 percent of college women and 88 percent of college men hooked up some time during college.[3] In a 2002–4 study of hooking up on a college campus, psychologist Elizabeth Paul of the College of New Jersey found that of 500 students surveyed, 75 percent reported hooking up, and about half of those who had hooked up had sex (the others did not report sexual intercourse). People who hooked up said that they rarely discussed sexual behaviors that they would participate in when they left the bar or party (or other location where they had met). This means they did not discuss protection, establish future relationship possibilities, or set sexual boundaries. In previous studies published by Paul, she found that the vast majority of people who had a hookup that involved sexual intercourse used condoms.[4] These results indicate that people may be more careful when engaging in sexual intercourse with unknown partners but less careful with those with whom they would like to start a relationship. A common belief that the participants in her study had was the presumption that women engaged in hookups to form a romantic relationship. However, hookups generally did not lead to romantic relationships; they were, in fact, temporary. Fewer than 25 percent of hookups in Dr. Paul's studies turned into relationships.

Paul is considered a national expert on hooking up and was interviewed by Anne Curry on the *Today Show* in 2004. Reflecting on her research in a press statement about the interview, Paul noted "that sexual experimentation among young adults is hardly novel but that these brief interactions have become more common in recent years and may be, to some degree, replacing traditional relationships." Paul said that many students in her focus groups believed that hookups offered an instant connection without the baggage that is associated with longer-term dating. She pointed out, however, that these encounters can have a significant downside, as well. There are obvious physical concerns, including sexually transmitted infections (STIs) and unplanned pregnancies. Psychologically, participants are often left to grapple with troubling emotions afterward. For Paul, one of the most distressing findings of her research "is that parents are afraid to broach the subject of hooking up with their children and students tend not to discuss bad 'hook-up' experiences with friends. Rather students internalize the negative feelings that arise from those instances."[5] It would be much better if young people learned from their hookup experiences; reflected on what occurred; discussed them with friends, family members, or health professionals; and made future decisions that were both mentally and physically healthy choices. Ultimately, the act of internalizing hookup experiences, particularly bad experiences, might prevent people from making better decisions in the future.

Paul also researched the conditions under which most hookups occurred. The most common activities to occur before hooking up included drinking alcohol, attending parties, dancing, flirting, or hanging out and talking. Large amounts of alcohol were a significant factor in determining whether a hookup led to actual intercourse compared to people who consumed smaller amounts of alcohol and hooked up with a person but did not have sex with him or her. Alcohol seems to be a significant factor in determining how far the hookup went.

Allison Caruthers, in her dissertation titled "'Hookups' and 'Friends with Benefits': Nonrelational Sexual Encounters as Contexts of Women's Normative Sexual Development," spent years at the University of Michigan studying the effect of hooking up on women's social and psychological development. There were three parts to Caruthers's study. She investigated the factors that made some women more prone to hooking up, if hooking up affected women's sexual health and well-being, and what the hookups meant to the women who participated in them. Caruthers wanted to see what factors affected emerging adult women's (late teens and early 20s) participation in hookups. She found that peer communication and perceptions of peer sexual behaviors were important factors in whether young women decided to participate in hooking up. Communication among friends that encouraged selflessness, self-objectification, and sexual exploration were each associated with women who had more hookups and started doing so at younger ages than women who did not have these kinds of communications with peer groups. Women who participated in hookups reported watching significantly more television in high school and overestimated the amount of sexual activity of their female peers compared to women who did not have sexual hookups.

Friends and parents of women who spoke to them about the importance of marriage and love seemed to deter women from hooking up with men. While Caruthers found that peer communication was the most important factor in determining hookup behaviors, parental communication about sex did influence the age at which women had their first hookup. In her sample of nearly 400 undergraduate students, the average age for the first hookup was around 16 years old. Parents who spoke to their daughters about the importance of marriage in sexual relationships seemed to delay the age of the first hookup experience. Interestingly, the content of messages did not matter as much as the number or volume of messages. Even women who had received messages that discouraged sexual exploration (such as "good girls do not engage in casual sexual encounters; they wait for marriage") were still more active than those who received fewer messages. Caruthers believes that hooking up may help women define boundaries and establish sexual identity and reconcile the different messages about sex that they receive from various important influences in their lives (from parents, the media, and peers).

It is noteworthy that the majority of studies and books about hooking up focus on women. In particular, popular culture discussions about hooking up, especially in the media, focus on women. This is probably due to sexual double standards of men and women, as discussed in chapter 3 of this book. Another reason is that society is simply more interested in monitoring and evaluating women's sexual experiences. The debate seems to revolve around whether hooking up is good or bad for women and whether it is good or bad for society. The effect that hooking up has on young men is largely ignored in this debate. However, these judgments seem to consider women, particularly young women who hook up, as deviant, lacking morals, or somehow falling short of societal expectations. As demonstrated in this chapter, research has provided mixed results about the effects of hooking up on women.

While conventional wisdom tells us that hooking up is bad for participants, especially women, Caruthers found otherwise. Conventional wisdom perpetuated by most journalists asserts that women hook up with men to (unsuccessfully) gain their attention and try to start relationships, to gain a false sense of sexual empowerment, or because they have low self-esteem or to avoid hurtful interpersonal relationships.[6] Some would even go as far as to call hooking up the breakdown of our society, and because women are participating in hookups, the very institution of marriage is going to fall apart.[7] Yes, in the short term, Caruthers found that women who hook up tend to have lower levels of well-being compared to women who do not; however, moderate levels of participation in hooking up had positive outcomes. Caruthers concluded that any negative effects or low levels of well-being were relatively short term. Moderate participation in hooking up resulted in women who had high levels of sexual assertiveness, sexual self-esteem, body comfort, and authenticity in close relationships. Overall, Caruthers believes that a little experimentation is good and that a little experimentation is much better for women than a lot of experimentation.[8] Moderation is key.

Last, Caruthers wanted to know what the experience of hooking up meant to women. Previous research on why women hook up, especially in college, found that women said they hooked up to start a long-term relationship, because they were drunk or using drugs at the time of the hookup, because they felt sexual desire, and/or because they wanted to explore and experiment with their sexuality. In addition, women may feel like emerging adulthood is the time to explore new partners and do something previously forbidden. Caruthers's research found that women made sense of hooking up in terms of three developmental tasks of emerging adulthood. First, women said hooking up helped them establish their own autonomy and independence. Second, women explored possible selves and different identities by hooking up. Third, women reported that hooking up helped them form emotionally intimate relationships with other people.

Due to the fact that hooking up is so widespread on college campuses, many people on campuses believe that others hook up a lot more than they really do. Individuals also believe that others are more comfortable hooking up than they really are. In fact, a study published in the *Journal of Sex Research* stated that both men and women reported less comfort with their perceived norm of hooking up than they believed was experienced by their peers.[9] Men showed a greater difference in their own ratings of comfort and their belief about other men's comfort hooking up. In other words, men greatly overestimated the level of other men's comfort hooking up. Women still overestimated the comfort levels of other women, but the divide was not as great. Interestingly, both men and women thought that the other gender was much more comfortable hooking up than they were in real life. Men thought women were more comfortable hooking up than they really were, and women thought men were more comfortable hooking up than they really were. This research is interesting given the high percentage of students who report engaging in hookups. Are they uncomfortable with their behaviors but going along with them because they think everyone else is doing it? Do they think they should be more comfortable hooking up than they are? One thing is certain: people surveyed in this study believed that others were more comfortable hooking up than themselves, especially men. Participants thought that everyone else was more comfortable than they were, not that some people would be more comfortable and some people less comfortable. Also, the study found that in real life, men are more comfortable hooking up than women.

FRIENDS WITH BENEFITS

The moniker "friends with benefits" implies in its name that two people care about each other and like each other. An exact definition of friendship is hard to pinpoint; however, friendships usually include the following characteristics: friendships are voluntary, personal relationships that are characterized by equality and mutual involvement, reciprocal liking, self-disclosure, and the provision of various kinds of support and care.[10] The name "friends with benefits" certainly does not have a negative connotation; rather, it conjures up the idea of two friends engaging in safe, friendly sex without the danger of sex with strangers or the emotional complications that accompany a relationship.

Throughout most of the literature on friendship development, it has been assumed that physical proximity has been a prerequisite for the formation of friendships—and to extend this line of thinking, friends with benefits. It can be assumed that friends-with-benefits sexual relationships (by definition) extend from a previously formed nonsexual friendship. The main places that people report making friends are in residential areas, work and school settings, and through social networks. For residential settings, neighbors and those who live the closest to people form the closest friendships. For example, people are more likely to become friends with people on the same floor of their apartment complex than with those on different floors. Work and school settings have been found to promote friendships because they provide great opportunities for interaction and contact. Also, many work tasks require cooperation, and numerous organizations encourage friendly behavior between workers. Social networks encourage friendship formation by introducing groups of friends to one another. When asked how they met their friends, most people report that they met them through other friends. A large part of whether a friendship will develop is dependant on whether a person's current social network will support (even encourage) the friendship, which will help a friendship grow. It is easy to see how friendships could blossom into sexual relationships because at the core of friendships are dyadic (between two people) relationships. However, with the advent of social networking through computer sources, scholars have been challenged to reconceptualize the assumption of proximity.

Despite how widespread the phenomenon of friends with benefits is, there has been relatively little study on it. Why do people participate in these relationships? Do they want to form more serious relationships? What do people talk about in terms of sex and safe sex? These are important questions to study. Most of the research on friends-with-benefits relationships has been completed on college campuses. All the studies show that between 50 and 60 percent of students reported having sex with a friend in the past.[11] According to Dr. Mikayla Hughes, a professor of communication at University of California, Davis, friends with benefits are different from other kinds of casual sexual encounters. Hookups are temporary, whereas friends with benefits tend to have more stability. This calls into question previous assumptions about the coexistence of sex and friendships, namely, that you cannot maintain a friendship with someone with whom you have had sex. Also, it defies popular culture beliefs that one individual will always want more of a relationship from this arrangement.

There was a recent study on teens and if being friends with benefits brought people closer together. For the majority, casual sex did not increase the closeness of a relationship. The results were published in an article in the *Journal of Adolescent Research* and reviewed the findings of the Toledo (Ohio) Adolescent Relationships Study and highlighted that many teens have casual sex.[12] About 30 percent of the 1,316 7th, 9th, and 11th graders had sexual intercourse. Sixty-one percent of sexually active teens have had sex with people whom they were not dating, mostly with friends or ex-boyfriends and/or ex-girlfriends. About half of the teens surveyed hoped that sex would lead to a more conventional dating relationship. Of the teens that did have sex outside of a dating relationship, there were no significant differences between boys' and girls' orientations toward relationships. The teens were asked how they felt after having casual sex with someone; 32 percent said that they felt closer to the person with whom they had sex, 52 percent reported that they felt like it did not change the relationship, and 15 percent said that it made them less close.

Just like in dating couples, the number one taboo topic in friends-with-benefits and casual sexual encounters is the actual state of the relationship. At first, people might think previous lovers or sexual history might be the most uncomfortable topic to discuss, but it is the status of the relationship. Will the casual hookup lead to anything more? Will the friends with benefits start dating publicly?

Communication patterns in friends-with-benefits relationships may share some patterns with romantic relationship development. For example, common topics that are considered taboo in romantic relationship development are the state of the relationship, expressing feelings about one another, sharing negative experiences that include discussing past abuse or rejections, past relationships including previous dating partners or marriages, sexual histories and preferences, and outside friendships.[13] Although I have not found any research indicating which of these patterns are followed, it makes sense that some of these topics may have been discussed previously in the friends-with-benefits relationship, particularly if people have the same group of friends. It is certainly much easier to find out information about a person's past dating experiences from mutual friends as compared to trying to find out information about a stranger that someone just started to date. However, I would imagine that relationship status and sharing feelings would be particularly avoided. Recall that in traditional romantic relationship development, the middle of the relationship (when the relationship is really escalating) is often the time of the least amount of personal disclosure and the highest period of topic avoidance because people do not want to do anything to jeopardize the relationship. Given this information, one would think that as friends-with-benefits relationships progress to romantic relationships, communication would be particularly guarded, even around the shared group of friends, so a person does not say anything to put the blossoming relationship in danger.

Another particularly important factor that may influence the transition of the friends-with-benefits relationship to a romantic close relationship is social networks. People who start out as friends often share a network of friends, which is different from the traditional linear dating relationship of two people who meet, become acquaintances, start to date, and then introduce one another to their friendship groups. Friends with benefits do not occur in a vacuum; rather, the networks of friends, particularly shared networks, may influence the trajectory to the relationship. Friends can either be a help or a hindrance. Here, if they choose to "go public," the couple will probably have a lot of relationship defining and explaining to do within their social network, which may be awkward. Reaction from the social network is important; research shows that romantic relationships that are supported by family and friends last longer and are more satisfying.[14] Some key transitioning points in friends-with-benefits relationships to romantic relationships include communicating about the relationship (labeling it), engaging in shared activities together (other than sexual activities), offering support in times of crisis, and going public with the relationship.

INTERNET DATING

Starting a relationship on the Internet has become a common way to meet someone. In the 1990s, when Internet dating first emerged, there was a stigma associated with it, fueled by negative media reports that highlighted people who were married and used the Internet to cheat, lied about their identities, or were sexual predators looking for prey. While there has not been a national survey of attitudes toward Internet dating, it is safe to say through anecdotal evidence that it has become mainstream, and much of the stigma, particularly for people 25 years and older, has been eliminated. It has been found that the Internet accelerates relationship development in many ways.[15] You certainly have the potential to meet a lot more people than in the small, daily world that most people inhabit. The Internet overcomes a lack of access to similar people and a lack of time that many people have in today's fast-paced world. First, people are less cautious about disclosure and, in particular, sexual disclosure because the Internet is relatively anonymous and rejection is much easier to face in this medium in comparison to a face-to-face encounter. People also tend to disclosure more because of perceived similarities. Sexual information may also be disclosed in a short amount of time if a person does not expect to meet in person or even interact with another person again on the Internet.

Second, the Internet removes some of the gating features that may inhibit the level of sexual disclosure in face-to-face encounters. Gating features include self-consciousness about physical characteristics, mannerisms, a lack of social skills, or personal traits such as shyness. Along this line, there is an absence of preconceived notions or stereotypes about people that all people have and make when they meet someone based on things like age, ethnicity, and attractiveness. People immediately and perhaps subconsciously tend to categorize people when they meet for the first time. As noted previously, first impressions are made within seconds of meeting someone and are significantly influenced by personal appearance. In a way, first impressions must be based on appearance because people just haven't had that much time to get to know someone. In the Internet world, first impressions are not as important.

Third, people tend to select Internet sites that already have people with similar interests, therefore accelerating the disclosure process. When you meet a stranger face-to-face, you do not know if she is interested in a relationship; however, there are many Internet sites with this specific goal in mind, taking out the ambiguity and allowing people to skip over some introductory knowledge-seeking behaviors. In fact, studies show that people are more likely to disclose their true or authentic selves much more quickly online than in person. For this reason alone, Internet dating is much more attractive to many people. In comparison, studies have shown that people liked those they met online first much more than if they had met them in person for the first time, which helps facilitate the initiation of close relationships over the Internet. It makes sense: most people want to be with someone who loves their true or authentic self, and if you can cut to the chase on the Internet in a safe way, then most people are likely to do so. Most close sexual relationships started over the Internet have been shown to be durable over time.

Putting all this together, chances are you may have more disclosure and meaningful communicating about sex over the Internet or in an Internet relationship because of the nature of skipping the small talk and because many of the barriers about saving face in naturally forming relationships do not exist.[16] In addition to the ones noted previously, most people meet through friends, at work, or in school. If you disclose personal sexual information to a person who you will have to see after the end of the hookup or relationship, you will think twice about disclosing. While people do not have real anonymity over the Internet (most people post their photographs and perhaps their professions; if someone tried hard enough, he could probably find out someone's identity), there is a perceived anonymity: people will not have to run into Internet connections at work, among friends, or at a local hangout such as the gym. Another thing that may facilitate sex talk is the fact that Internet communication is not instant. Much of the awkwardness of initiating a topic and then having to wait for that person to respond, attempting to read their nonverbal cues, and so on, can be intimidating. However, with the Internet, much of this is removed: people do not expect an immediate reply, and people can take time forming their e-mails in long, well thought out statements that are often proofread. There is ample opportunity to fully explain your beliefs and personality in a polished, planned manner. In turn, the person can read the e-mail, think about it, and reply in kind. All the awkwardness of face-to-face communication—the long pauses, ums, and the need for an immediate response—are removed. There is much more control over conversations on the Internet, despite the main flaw of delayed immediacy.

COMMUNICATION STYLES AND SPEED DATING

Speeding dating is a fairly new way to meet people; less than 10 years ago, it was invented by Rabbi Yaacov Deyo in Los Angles as a way for Jewish singles to get to meet one another with the purpose of dating in mind. The social atmosphere at speed-dating events is much more like a singles bar or a party rather than a traditional date but is unique in several ways. Speed dating is different from dating in that the durations of the dates are significantly different; the atmosphere is social, lively, and nonintimate; and any bad date is easy to get out of, with no excuses or awkward good-byes. Unlike a club or party, certain assumptions are made about the participants in speed dating, namely, that the participants are romantically available and interested in meeting someone. Plus, people do not have to worry about awkward introductions or pickup lines or need a great deal of confidence. One of the most interesting findings of research on speed dating is that in general, people make accurate inferences and judgments about a person after a short amount of time. It seems that people do not need a prolonged, romantic date to determine if they are romantically interested and attracted to a person. If there were fewer stigmas attached to alternative forms of dating, such as speed dating, they would be used much more because they are so efficient.

Another interesting thing about speed dating, and even meeting some-one in person, is that the prior judgments and beliefs about what people think they are looking for in a partner may not be accurate. For example, in a study, people were asked before a dating event to list the character-istics that they believed to be most important to them: earning potential was one for women and physical attractiveness was one for men. How-ever, after the speed-dating event, when asked about whom people se-lected and why, it became clear that these criteria were not important.[17] Often people cannot account for sexual chemistry and attraction.

One thing that both Internet dating and speed dating have in common is the ability to pass on the societal dictates that state that new conver-sations should be superficial and that if we choose to intensify the rela-tionship, the conversations become gradually more intimate. Indeed, if, on a date, a person skipped over the normal protocol of asking about someone's drive (or walk) over or the weather that day, and jumped to something such as what the person was looking for in a romantic rela-tionship, it would probably be a bad sign to the other person. He or she might be thinking, "Slow down! Is this person desperate or what?" How-ever, the ability to cut to the chase and have informed, direct communica-tion with someone else is also beneficial in that it saves time but allows people to express their authentic selves and not have to worry about the timing of letting people in.

SAFE SEX: THE TALK IN A CASUAL RELATIONSHIP

What kind of information do people talk about when it comes to sex-ual health? A study by communication scholar Rebecca Cline[18] showed that the most commonly discussed topics included sexual history (dis-cussions about the type of people a person was with previously) and gen-eral conversations about sexual health and clinical topics (discussing how infections are transmitted sexually); a small percentage (10%) discussed intended condom use. In another study by communication expert Tim Edgar, people most often talked more indirectly about sexual health. For example, in his study, most people asked about sexual experience and commitment. Around 77 percent asked about the number of previ-ous partners a person had, 64 percent asked about the last time some-one had sex, and 55 percent inquired whether someone had a current sexual partner. Whereas 66 percent of people did address sexual health concerns by asking how someone felt about using condoms with a previous sexual partner, 44 percent asked if someone had a STI. All these conversations were marked with self-disclosures, joking, and indirect and direct questions.[19]

Another study by Cline examined the extent to which heterosexual college students talked with their sexual partners about AIDS.[20] She asked 588 undergraduate students about the nature of discussions about AIDS. Cline found that 63.6 percent of the participants had discussed AIDS with a partner, but 20.7 percent had discussed topics related to safe sex, and only 6.3 percent discussed useful means of AIDS prevention. This study was completed in 1992, when AIDS was a much scarier topic and got more media coverage. It would be interesting to see how many current college students discuss AIDS, now that it is not at the forefront of STI fears. However, these results are still important because they show that talking with a partner about AIDS does not necessarily increase AIDS prevention measures. In other words, we can assume that many people may talk about diseases and the consequences of sexual activity, but that does not translate into 100 percent effective safe-sex measures. Indeed, few people report using condoms every time they have intercourse, which is necessary to prevent STIs, particularly in casual sex.

Effective communication skills in women have been positively related to condom use. What does effective communication mean? And how do we ask our sexual partners about sex-related information? Even in close relationships, people consider sex a taboo topic.[21] Therefore many people resort to passive sexual information–seeking strategies, particularly people who are at the beginning stages of relationship development or involved in nonrelational sex. The most common way people determine the sexual health of a potential partner is by observing how they look or where they are socializing. For example, one study found that people determined that a partner was risky if she dressed "slutty," was at a bar, or was older than they were. This kind of decision making is based on *relational radar*, a feeling or impression people get about how risky a sexual encounter would be. Ironically, other studies showed that safe-sex behaviors, such as carrying a condom in a wallet or having access to a condom in the bedroom, communicated a negative impression of a person rather than that person being sexual responsible. It is very difficult to engage in active information seeking without talking with the person. Some of the other ways people reported finding out sexual information other than having directly asked a person was by asking a third party or going through the person's personal belongings for sexual health information. These are not that effective because asking third parties about a person's sexual health may be awkward and of limited usefulness. Also, most people do not leave information about their sexual health lying around, if they have any information at all. The only other way to seek information is to communicate directly with the person.

BARRIERS TO SAFE-SEX COMMUNICATION

In a recent study, female, heterosexual, undergraduate students were interviewed about the health-protective sexual communication that did or did not occur with their most recent sexual partners prior to first intercourse.[22] The narratives derived from this qualitative study provided insight into the context and extent of health-protective sexual communication occurring prior to intercourse, the perceived barriers and facilitators to health-protective sexual communication, and the strategies used to initiate such discussions. Sexual communication has been identified as one of the key components in understanding the interpersonal interactions that facilitate or impede sexual health–protective behaviors, including condom use. Despite the importance of communicating with one's sexual partner, researchers have found that the initiation of sexual health–related discussions is difficult for most people and that the seeming reluctance to talk about these issues appears to be fueled by numerous perceived personal and relationship barriers, including (but not limited to) lack of comfort, feelings of awkwardness and ineptness with sexual health–related discussions, lack of effective communication skills, lack of belief in the ability to communicate, use of drugs and alcohol, expected negative outcomes of having such discussions, fear of embarrassment, and shame. The possible negative relationship implications of discussing sexual health issues with a partner are among the most commonly cited reasons for people to avoid such communication. The reasons for this avoidance are that people do not want to threaten their relationships or ruin the romance, intimacy, and spontaneity in their relationships. Also, they fear the potential partner's anticipated reaction and the fact that asking implies a lack of trust in a potential partner.

Another thing is clear from most of the studies, regardless of age group. Many of the relational and sexual terms people use today are deliberately ambiguous. If you are asking about your sexual partner's previous sexual history and the person refers to hooking up with someone last weekend, it could mean any range of sexual activities. It makes it even more awkward to talk about sex because a person may have to press for specific details before they will be provided. As we learned in chapter 1, concrete language is much better than abstract language. Also, because there is ambiguity in even basic terms, such as *dating*, people may be unclear about the status of their sexual relationships and could therefore be more cautious about sex talk, not wanting to jeopardize the relationship or to talk about commitment issues too soon. Many people prefer indirect communication because there are higher levels of ambiguity, allowing them to save face if things do not go well. Direct communication often demands a response, just as explicit requests for information about sexual activity or relationship status demand a response. It short, direct or explicit communication puts people on the spot to respond. During sexual and/or relational initiation, each person is negotiating levels of attraction, self-disclosure, and interest.

Another significant barrier to sex talk is the fact that so much communication around sex is nonverbal, which makes talking about safer sex difficult. Because people rarely talk about their sexual intentions, especially in casual relationships, it is hard to talk about sexual history and taking precautions. Most people negotiate sex nonverbally, and if a condom is used, many times, it is because one person pulls out a condom and puts it on the man, without even saying a word.

SEX TALK AND CASUAL SEX

"Despite the effectiveness of consistent and careful condom use, many sexually active Americans are still engaging in unprotected sexual activities."[23] Seth Noar, sexual communication expert from the University of Kentucky, and his colleagues found that length and type of relationship are significant predictors in terms of condom use.[24] However, Noar contends that when it comes to safe sex and disclosure about STIs, there is only a perception that communication about STI status is better in close relationships. In reality, being in a close relationship may make it harder to get at someone's real STI status.

Richard de Visser, from the Australian Research Center in Sex, Health, and Society, found that condom use is more habitual in main or close relationships as compared to those that are more casual relationships because people do not have to negotiate condom use every time in a close relationship as compared to different partners in a casual sexual encounter.[25] Also, a lot of research shows that alcohol is involved in casual, nonrelational sex, which makes it more difficult to communicate effectively and engage in safe-sex practices. However, a common finding in studies of heterosexual young adults is that condom use is more likely with casual partners than with regular partners because people do not trust one another in a casual encounter. Many times people in close relationships switch to oral birth control or take more chances when having sex. In 2001, de Visser completed a study involving 103 heterosexual men and women who completed a condom use diary for a period of up to six months. He found that condom use during sexual encounters with regular partners was mainly determined by established patterns of behavior. In contrast, condom use with casual partners was determined by the interaction between the sexual partners during the encounter and was not influenced by the attitudes and beliefs of the individual. De Visser's findings are important when it comes to communication skills as the findings suggest that condom use with casual partners may be increased when people are provided with the skills and confidence necessary to negotiate condom use. For people in close, regular relationships, it is essential to establish a routine pattern of condom use that is appropriate for the levels of risk to which the partners are exposed. It is important to establish safe-sex routines at the beginning of a relationship because this will set the pattern for the rest of the relationship.

While I stress that meaningful communication about sex is essential, the fact is that joking can release tension, serve as verbal foreplay, and decrease inhibitions to talk about safer sex. There is definitely a place for humor in sexual relationships, particularly at the beginning of a relationship, when one person (or both) is trying to establish a pattern of condom use and safe sex.

The research in the chapter presented two equally compelling research findings. First, people are more likely to use condoms in casual sexual encounters because they do not trust or know the other person. In contrast, other research has concluded that people are more likely to use condoms in close sexual relationships because once they have become established as birth control, there is no need to constantly renegotiate their use, whereas in casual sex, there is constant negotiation (and a chance a person will fail to successfully negotiate use). Either way, it is important to be protected during a casual encounter. We also know from gender roles that most people leave it up to the man to talk about or provide and use condoms, whereas most people feel that women are ultimately held responsible for any consequences of sex and are supposed to nurture relationships. It is important for both men and women to be aware of these gender roles and overcome them; both parties need to be actively involved in protective measures. If it helps, readers could even joke about the gender roles and what is supposed to happen. Humor goes a long way in casual encounters because they are supposed to be lighter compared to sex in more serious relationships.

Another thing that people can do is discuss or set limits on the sexual activities that they are comfortable with before they leave a place with someone, or at least, they can do this mentally. It is difficult when someone asks "hey, do you want to go someplace more quiet?" or "do you want to go back to my place?" to then say immediately, "Sure, but we can only engage in oral sex, that is my limit" or "Sure, but I will only have sex with a condom . . . if it gets that far." This indeed would be awkward. But think about how awkward, difficult, and even dangerous it would be once you are with that person, in the middle of things, naked, and in bed.

Friends-with-benefits relationships involve unique challenges to communication about sex. First, people do not want to jeopardize the relationship by asking uncomfortable questions such as "am I the only person you are having sex with now?" "how much unprotected sex have you had?" "have you ever been tested for a STI?" "would you be willing to get tested?" Questions like this and events such as getting tested are usually reserved for close romantic relationships; however, friends with benefits fall somewhere in between the one-night stand or casual sex and a close relationship. Usually, there are repeated sexual encounters and interpersonal interactions between sexual episodes. While questions such as these may seem like they push the "where is this relationship going?" question, simply preface the conversation with something like, "Look, this is not a conversation about us or the state of the relationship, this is about health. We need to discuss these issues in order to protect us both and I need you to tell me the truth."

IMPLICATIONS FOR SEX TALK

- Do not be afraid to talk to your parents or children about hooking up. Parents should be talking about hooking up with their teenage and young adult children.
- Try to be more forthcoming about your hookup experiences with friends. People often keep negative hookup experiences to themselves, which can increase the negative effects of the hookup.
- Realize that people are not hooking up as much as you think and are not as comfortable with hooking up as you think. As shown in the research, both men and women overestimate the comfort levels of hooking up of others. You can talk about this with the person with whom you are hooking up and use it as entrée into a discussion about safe-sex behaviors.

- Realize that it is more myth than reality that hookups lead to relationships and that women are hooking up as a means to start a relationship. By participants laying the cards on the table, so to speak, it can also open up the discussion to health issues and issues of sexual comfort (likes and dislikes).

- Understand that alcohol is a significant factor in whether a hookup will lead to sex. If you do not want to have sex or unprotected sex during a hookup, watch your level of alcohol intake, ask a friend to watch out for you, or talk directly to your hookup about your limits.

NOTES

1. Edward Herold, Eleanor Maticka-Tyndale, and Dawn Mewhinney, "Predicting Intentions to Engage in Casual Sex," *Journal of Social and Personal Relationships* 15 (1998): 502–16.

2. Michael Cunningham and Anita Barbee, "Prelude to a Kiss: Nonverbal Flirting, Opening Gambits, and Other Communication Dynamics in the Initiation of Romantic Relationships," in *Handbook of Relationship Initiation*, ed. Susan Sprecher, Amy Wenzel, and John Harvey (New York: Psychology Press, 2008).

3. T. A. Lambert, A. S. Kahn, and K. J. Apple, "Pluralistic Ignorance and Hooking Up," *Journal of Sex Research* 40, no. 2 (2003).

4. Elizabeth L. Paul and Kristen A. Hayes, "The Casualties of 'Casual' Sex: A Qualitative Exploration of the Phenomenology of College Students' Hookups," *Journal of Social and Personal Relationships* 19 (2002). Elizabeth L. Paul, Brian McManus, and Allison Hayes, "'Hookups': Characteristics and Correlates of College Students' Spontaneous and Anonymous Sexual Experiences," *Journal of Sex Research* 37 (2000).

5. The College of New Jersey, "*Today Show, Newsweek* Feature Research of TCNJ Professor," press release, http://www.tcnj.edu/~pa/news/2004/Beth Paul.htm.

6. Allison S. Caruthers, "'Hookups' and 'Friends with Benefits': Nonrelational Sexual Encounters as Contexts of Women's Normative Sexual Development" (UMI Microform 3192595, ProQuest Information & Learning, 2006), 80.

7. See Laura Sessions Stepp, *Unhooked: How Young Women Pursue Sex, Delay Love, and Lose at Both* (New York: Riverhead Books, 2007).

8. Caruthers, "'Hookups' and 'Friends with Benefits,'" 159.

9. Tracy A Lambert, Arnold S Kahn, and Kevin J Apple, "Pluralistic Ignorance and Hooking Up," *Journal of Sex Research* 40, no. 2 (2003): 129–33.

10. Beverley Fehr, "Friendship Formation," in *Handbook of Relationship Initiation*, ed. Susan Sprecher, Amy Wenzel, and John Harvey (New York: Psychology Press, 2008).

11. Mikayla Hughes, Kelly Morrison, and Kelli Jean K. Asada, "What's Love Got to Do with It? Exploring the Impact of Maintenance Rules, Love Attitudes, and Network Support on Friends with Benefits Relationships," *Western Journal of Communication* 69 (2005).

12. Wendy D. Manning, Peggy C. Giordano, and Monica A. Longmore, "Hooking Up: The Relationship Contexts of 'Nonrelationship' Sex," *Journal of Adolescent Research* 21, no. 5 (2006).

13. Laura Guerrero and Paul Mongeau, "On Becoming 'More Than Friends': The Transition from Friendship to Romantic Relationship," in *Handbook of Relationship Initiation*, ed. Susan Sprecher, Amy Wenzel, and John Harvey (New York: Psychology Press, 2008), 186.

14. Ibid., 180.

15. Valerian Derlega, Barbara Winstead, and Kathryn Greene, "Self-Disclosure and Starting a Close Relationship," in *Handbook of Relationship Initiation*, ed. Susan Sprecher, Amy Wenzel, and John Harvey (New York: Psychology Press, 2008), 166.

16. Katelyn McKenna, "MySpace or Your Place: Relationship Initiation and Development of the Wired and Wireless World," in *Handbook of Relationship Initiation*, ed. Susan Sprecher, Amy Wenzel, and John Harvey (New York: Psychology Press, 2008).

17. Paul Eastwick and Eli Finkel, "Speed-Dating: A Powerful and Flexible Paradigm for Studying Romantic Relationship Initiation," in *Handbook of Relationship Initiation*, ed. Susan Sprecher, Amy Wenzel, and John Harvey (New York: Psychology Press, 2008).

18. Rebecca Welch Cline, K. Freeman, and S. Johnson, "Talk among Sexual Partners About AIDS: Interpersonal Communication for Risk Reduction or Risk Enhancement?" *Health Communication* 4 (1992).

19. Timothy Edgar, Vicki Friemuth, S. Hammond, D. McDonald, and Edgar Fink, "Strategic Sexual Communication: Condom Use Resistance and Response," *Health Communication* 4 (1992).

20. Rossella E. Nappi, Kathrin Wawra, and Sonja Schmitt, "Hypoactive Sexual Desire Disorder in Postmenopausal Women," *Gynecological Endocrinology* 22, no. 6 (2006).

21. Walid Afifi and Alysa Lucas, "Information Seeking in the Initial Stages of Relational Development," in *Handbook of Relationship Initiation*, ed. Susan Sprecher, Amy Wenzel, and John Harvey (New York: Psychology Press, 2008), 143.

22. Jennifer Cleary, Richard Barhman, Terry MacCormack, and Ed Herold, "Discussing Sexual Health with a Partner: A Qualitative Study with Young Women," *Canadian Journal of Human Sexuality* 11 (2002).

23. Mike Allen, Tara Emmers-Sommer, and Tara Crowell, "Couples Negotiating Safer Sex Behaviors: A Meta-Analysis of the Impact of Conversation and Gender," in *Interpersonal Communication Research: Advances through Meta-Analysis*, ed. Raymond W. Preiss, Barbara Mae Gayle, and Nancy A. Burrell (Mahwah, NJ: Lawrence Erlbaum Associates, 2002), 263.

24. Seth Noar, Rick Zimmerman, and Katherine Atwood, "Safer Sex and Sexually Transmitted Infections from a Relationship Perspective," in *The Handbook of Sexuality in Close Relationships*, ed. John Harvey, Amy Wenzel, and Susan Sprecher (Mahwah, NJ: Lawrence Erlbaum Associates, 2005).

25. Richard de Visser, Anthony Smith, Chris E. Rissel, Juliet Richters, and Andrew E. Grulich, "Sex in Australia: Safer Sex and Condom Use Among a Representative Sample of Adults," *Australian and New Zealand Journal of Public Health* 27, no. 12 (2007): 223–29.

CHAPTER 6

Relationship Initiation and Communication about Sex in First-Time and Dating Relationships

"Oh man, the balancing act needed to ask a girl out is brutal. I feel like I am walking on a tightrope. I have to seem as interested, but not too interested, friendly, but not too innocuous, and desirable, but not too sexual. You women ask for too much. I cannot be direct and let someone know I like her. I have to wait for her to get the hint before I can even start flirting with her. Also, I know you women are judging men. If I compliment a woman on her appearance, I run the risk of seeming like I want something, rather than just giving her a compliment. Or a girl just thinks I am after a hookup or something short term. The long-term stuff is really hard to manage," Jim said. Jim is a 30 something guy who was back on the dating market after his four-year relationship with his girlfriend ended about six months ago. He was lamenting his problems to his friend Sarah.

"I know, I know. It is not easy for women either. I was just reading a study that said that people think it is OK to lie to get a date when the person is really attractive. The more attractive someone is, the more acceptable it is to lie. I mean, how are we supposed to know if a guy is interested in something more long term? Some people say it's when a guy starts disclosing things like his financial status, things that would make him a better catch. But guys can't appear too anxious or we immediately think you are trying to deceive us for some reason. History has taught us to be careful," Sarah lamented.

"The ball is in your court, you know. You get one chance and if you shoot us down, men don't really try again. Most men only ask once and then move on. There is only so much rejection a guy can take. And we know from history that once a woman says no, it's not worth pursuing," Jim stated.

"Yeah, it's a lot of pressure, being hit on. No, seriously, I am not kidding. Not only do we have to determine if we really are being hit on, but we have like a split second or something to decide what your motives are and if we are interested. And we don't even have a lot of information. It's not like we can sit there and play 20 questions when we are hit on or something. Let's face it, we can only decide on two things, how attractive the guy is and how he communicates, you know, how he talks to us," Sarah replied. "Negotiating the start of a relationship is not easy for men or women."

INTRODUCTION

Most relationships do not move along a linear continuum; we meet someone, date, fall in love, and have sex in a nice, orderly manner. Sexual relationships, in particular, do not follow a linear path. Rather, people might meet, have sex, then fall in love. It is important to keep in mind that relationships develop differently. Some researchers and people believe that relationships develop through a progressive tract and that there are certain landmarks that each relationship passes through. This progress is linear. Dr. Steve Duck wants people consider a different approach to relationship development. He suggests that relationships could be like frogs, which develop from tadpoles by growing legs and enlarging themselves. A relationship is not going somewhere, but growing somehow. Or he suggests that we consider an insect metaphor; relationships metamorphose from egg to larva to pupa to nymph. Each stage is developed from the previous form, but it is completely different and transformed from the original form and each subsequent form. Here relationships grow to form new, unrecognizable shapes as they develop.[1] Even though most relationships do not develop in a linear manner, researchers found that people whose relationships developed in the way they thought relationships should typically develop had higher rates of relational satisfaction.[2] People did not have to agree with their partners on how a relationship should develop to have high rates of relational satisfaction. Each person may have different ideas about how a relationship should develop. But before we get to the development of relationships, we have to start at the beginning. What attracts us to other people? What are most people looking for in a mate? What role does communication play in the attraction process?

RESEARCH ON ATTRACTION, COMMUNICATION STYLE, AND PARTNER PREFERENCES: DO BIRDS OF A FEATHER FLOCK TOGETHER? OR DO OPPOSITES ATTRACT?

So what attracts us to certain people? What role does communication play in the attraction process? People have unique preferences for certain characteristics in romantic partners based on individual and cultural influences. These preferences can be expected to guide choices in relational initiation and growth. It is commonly accepted that proximity, similarity, physical attractiveness, complementarity, quality of communication, and possession of resources are precursors of attraction.[3] Proximity refers to the closeness and availability of people. Proximity is important because we have the greatest opportunities to get to know the people with whom we live, play, and work. We tend to like the people we know because we can predict their behaviors better than those of a complete stranger. There is less uncertainty with people known to us. Conventional wisdom tells us that proximity is usually the most common reason that people become romantically or sexually attracted to one another. Numerous research also indicates that proximity determines who our closest friends are, as well.

The Internet is slowly changing how we view proximity because it allows for more opportunities for people to find similar people. *Similarity* refers to the idea that we want people who are like us. The *matching hypothesis* predicts that although people are attracted to the most physically attractive people, they will date and marry people who are similar to them in physical attractiveness.[4] Researchers predict that most people, if asked to describe their ideal mates, would present a mirror image of themselves: similar nationality, race, abilities, physical characteristics, intelligence, and attitudes. *Complementarity*, on the other hand, suggests that we are attracted to dissimilar others. We fall in love with people who have characteristics that we may not possess but admire in others. So, for example, the shy introvert may be attracted to an outgoing extrovert.

Both complementarity and matching theory are widely believed by many to be the most important elements of attraction, and both have some level of validity. However, the dominant line of thinking regarding interpersonal relationships and attraction is that people with similar interests are attracted to one another and talk (conversations) is used to uncover those similarities. Steve Duck, a communication researcher from the University of Iowa and an expert on interpersonal relation-ships, believes otherwise.[5] He believes that when two people meet and start to date, the success of the relationship is not dependent on whether they have similar personalities; rather, it is based on how they talk to each other. Therefore it is important to pay attention to how we say things and respond to what others say to us. Duck believes that rela-tional maintenance contains two elements: the first is strategic planning for the continuance of the relationship, and the second is the light-hearted allowance of the relationship to continue by means of the every-day interactions and conversations that make the relationship what it is. The kind of relationship that develops largely depends on how peo-ple manage the relationship as they talk. Early in his career, Duck did studies that showed that communication quality increases interpersonal attraction. Attraction is an important predictor of relationship initiation, intensification, and preservation. Therefore quality of communication can be seen as a significant dynamic in both initial attraction and deter-mining if the relationship will take off and become serious.

Anthropologist Helen Fisher, from Rutgers University in New Jersey, has made a career out of studying romance and love. Based on the re-search she completed with neuroscientists, she believes "that the basic human emotions and motivations arise from distinct circuits or systems of neural activity. Among these neural systems, humanity has evolved three distinctly different yet interrelated brain systems for courtship, mating, reproduction and parenting. These are lust, romantic love, and male/female attachment."[6] In a study of human sexual arousal, neuro-scientists took scans of the brain using magnetic resonance imagining. When each of the three different types of systems was activated, spe-cific and distinct networks of brain activation were recorded for lust, romantic love, and male-female attachment. This shows that the dif-ferences in lust, love, and attachment are not just psychological, but physiological. Researchers have also established a chemical link be-tween romantic love and lust; romantic love triggers the drive to pursue sex. Lust is characterized by the yearning for sexual gratification and is linked to the androgens in men and women. Androgens are male sex hormones that are found in both men and women. Romantic love has been characterized by elation, increased energy, mood swings, focused attention, obsessive thinking, desire to be reunited with a beloved part-ner, and a powerful motivation to win a preferred mate. Male-female attachment is also known as compassionate love. This is characterized by the maintenance of proximity, affectionate gestures, expressions of calm and contentment when with a partner, and anxiety over separation when apart. Each of these brain systems for loving produces different thoughts, ways of thinking, and behaviors and requires different communication approaches. For example, in compassionate love situations where one is talking about sex, partner feelings and consideration should be of great importance, whereas in lustful situations, health-protective behaviors should be at the forefront.

We know that people look for different things in different kinds of relationships. Studies have examined different types of people that we seek in friendships versus romantic relationships and what people look for in short-term versus long-term relationships. One study examined the degree to which different characteristics are desired in a casual sex partner, dating partner, marriage partner, same-sex friend, or opposite-sex friend.[7] In general, the study found that most people preferred others who were warm and kind, had high levels of expressivity and openness, and a good sense of humor in all types of relationships (even casual sex partners). These characteristics were highly desired and valued all in types of relationships and are clearly intrinsic rather than extrinsic attributes such as wealth and beauty. But when it came to differences people look for in sexual relationships, people had higher expectations than in their friendships, particularly same-sex friendships. Most people felt that it was more important to find someone with higher levels of physical attractiveness, social status attributes, and warmth, expressiveness, humor, and intelligence in a romantic/sexual partner than in a friend.

Although people stated that they wanted casual sex partners to have all the qualities that they were looking for in a long-term relationship, they were willing to settle for less when it came down to it. Interestingly, people also indicated that they had different standards for same-sex and opposite-sex friendships. The standards seemed to be higher for opposite-sex friendships compared to same-sex friendships, where most people said they preferred higher levels of physical attractiveness, social status, and dispositional/personality attributes from opposite-sex friends than from same-sex friends. Last, they found that women were more attuned than men to their own value as a partner and how this value influences the kind of partner that they could potentially attract and retain.

Another study looked at women's and men's desired characteristics in partners for typical short-term and long-term relationships.[8] For the purpose of the study, *short term* was defined as dating someone more than once without an expectation of a short- or long-term relationship, and *long term* was defined as dating someone for a long time with the possibility, but not certainty, of marriage. Not surprisingly, both women and men were more discriminating when selecting a long-term rather than a short-term relationship partner. As previously stated, people may desire the same characteristics in short-term relationships but settle for less. However, this study found that women and men desire different characteristics in people for short-term relationship partners and long-term relationship partners. True to stereotype, this research study found that men believed reproductive-value characteristics, such as physical attractiveness, were important in women, and women stated that high resource-acquisition abilities, such as earning capacity, were important for potential male partners. While there were significant differences between men and women in their desired characteristics in short- and long-term relationship partners, there were many similarities in what they sought, such as the desire for children in long-term partners and an exciting personality in short-term and long-term partners.

Prior to 1985, most relationship initiation and attraction theories focused on the concepts of costs and benefits (we will be attracted to people who provide us the greatest rewards and benefits with minimal costs). So if we find someone similar to us, we will be more attracted to him because he will reward us for our thoughts and ideas rather than punish us. Everything could conceptually fit into these two categories of cost or benefit. When the punishments or costs became greater than the rewards, then people ended the relationship. The two modern theories that most attraction experts focus on are evolutionary theory and attachment theory.

Throughout this book, evolutionary theory has been mentioned. One of the most famous researchers in this area is Dr. David Buss. In the most basic sense, evolutionary theorists believe that we are attracted to people who have qualities that enhance reproductive success. People become attracted to those they believe will increase their chances of the successful conception, birth, and survival of their offspring. Attraction is driven by an internal conscious or even subconscious drive to find the best mate for reproduction. A typical study of evolutionary theory comprises the series of research studies that Michael Cunningham and colleagues published on the facial features of women.[9] Cunningham asked male college students to rate the attractiveness of a group of women in photographs. Half of the women were college seniors, and the other half were international beauty contestants. Not surprisingly, the international beauty contestants received higher ratings of attractiveness. Dr. Cunningham then ran statistical tests to see what kinds of features made someone more attractive than others. He found that facial characteristics that were associated with neonatal features such as large eyes and a large mouth relative to facial area; mature features such as chin width; and expressive features such as smile width made women more attractive to men. Cunningham believes these facial features predict the perception of fertility and health.

Another study found that men prefer average faces rather than individual faces, meaning that men have an aversion for faces different from the norm.[10] However, in evolutionary theory, everything is not based on looks alone. Men gain their attractiveness through their social status and resources and dominance. These characteristics and behaviors, from an evolutionary standpoint, make men seem more healthy and able to provide for offspring. Dominance, however, is a behavior and not an innate feature. In a study about attraction and dominance, researchers found that females were more attracted to dominant men (men who in the experiment used dominant behaviors such as direct eye contact or a relaxed seating position) compared to men using nondominant behaviors.[11] Interestingly, dominance increased men's attraction but not likeability scores.

The other approach to attractiveness is based more on social construction and culture and says social factors such as personality, situation, timing, and so forth make some people more attractive than others. A typical study in this area could be a famous one done on the attractiveness of women who are in a bar at closing time. Different studies have researched how men rate women's attractiveness over the course of an evening at a bar or nightclub. The studies found that girls get prettier at closing time. In one study done by Dr. Madey, researchers asked men to rate the attractiveness of women at a bar three different times at night: at 10:00 P.M., midnight, and 1:30 A.M.[12] Indeed, attractiveness ratings went up for the women remaining in the bar. Another fascinating component to attraction theory is that beauty is not simply external and objective; beauty is also in the eye of the beholder. Men and women report reciprocal liking, personality, physical appearance, kindness and warmth, fun, caring, and motivation as the most frequent types of romantic attractors.[13] In another study, men and women rated the main five dimensions of personality they thought were essential for attraction. The five factors were extroversion, agreeableness, conscientiousness, emotional stability, and openness. For example, for both men and women, people who were rated as agreeable were viewed as significantly more attractive than those who were disagreeable. Interestingly, the measure of agreeableness is also internal to the person making the judgment. For example, "persons high in agreeableness say that they like more people, including traditional targets of prejudice, than do other peers. Persons low in agreeableness (particularly men) show lower levels of attraction and actively discriminate against out-group women (in this case, overweight women) at the initiation phase of a relationship."[14] People who are likeable and agreeable find more people to be likeable and agreeable, as well.

In a study by Steve Duck and Susan Sprecher, the perceived quality of communication on a first date was tested to see how important it was on dating and friendship attraction, on dating partners' desire to see each other again, and on continuation of the relationship.[15] The importance of partner's physical attractiveness and similarity were also considered. In a scenario where strangers were set up and sent on a date, all the singles judged the quality of communication to be high and experienced at least some attraction for their partner, but only 10 of 70 couples contacted at follow-up had been on a second date. Not surprisingly, perceived physical attractiveness and similarity were the strongest predictors of romantic attraction; however, the quality of communication was related to attraction and to desire to see the partner again. The importance of quality of communication was greater for women than for men and greater for friendship attraction than for romantic attraction.

RELATIONSHIP INITIATION
AND PICKUP LINES

Like the old saying goes, "you only get to make a first impression once." Nothing could be more true. Whether you are deciding how to describe yourself in a paragraph for an online dating site, being introduced to a potential partner by a friend, or approaching a stranger, the first impression is important. People first approach someone when they are attracted to her for some reason and want to see if there is mutual interest. Most people gather enough information within the first minute of conversation with a stranger to determine whether the target person is someone who is suitable and interesting enough to pursue a romantic association.[16] Generally, the first few minutes of interaction with a stranger are question laden. One study showed that people ask around 22 questions in the first five minutes of an interaction.[17] There are three ways that people usually seek information about a potential date or hookup: through question asking, self-disclosure, or relaxing the person. Interrogation or question asking is the most direct form of information gathering and is also commonly regarded as the least appropriate and most intrusive by both men and women. Another strategy is to use self-disclosure to encourage the person to reciprocate with his own disclosures. The idea in relaxing the person is that through nonverbal and verbal behavior, the target becomes comfortable enough to become vulnerable and disclose personal information. Before anyone gets to the first five minutes of a conversation, however, she has to start the conversation, and that is why opening lines are so important.

Opening lines are critical in that they may determine whether an initial encounter goes any further. Researchers found that there are three kinds of pickup lines: the cute-flippant line, the direct approach, and the innocuous approach. The cute-flippant approach involves a person who wants to appear witty or humorous, uses glib statements, and/or uses cliché pickup lines. The direct approach usually involves someone introducing himself, making a blatant statement of attraction, or presenting an invitation to participate in a joint activity such as "Do you want to dance?" or "Can I buy you a cup of coffee?" The innocuous approach is a harmless initial contact (perhaps a statement about the weather or a request for the time of day), where someone can test to see if a person is willing to engage in conversation. In general, men respond to any kind of pickup line, whereas numerous studies show that women overwhelmingly prefer innocuous initial interactions.[18] This is not surprising because overall, women are more discriminating when it comes to potential sexual partners than men. Researchers found that women have higher standards for sex than a single date, whereas men had a higher standard for a date than a sexual encounter.[19] In other words, women will go on a date with a larger number of people and have a lower overall standard for a date than men but are more discriminating when it comes to sex. Men would be more willing to have sex with a larger number of women than they would ask on a date. We can assume this is because men perceive that they may actually have to pay for the date, or perhaps a date is a greater investment of time and energy.

Despite the fact that males and females are dictated by the cultural script that men should be the one to make the first move, females often control the early phases of courtship.[20] For example, a male must wait for a female to show interest before he can approach her. From a male's point of view, if he attempts to approach a female who has not given him signs of sexual interest, then he is unlikely to be successful. Women are much more likely to be approached when they display solicitous behaviors, including smiling, eye contact, glancing around the room, solitary dancing, laughing, and the ever popular hair flipping.

LIFE ISN'T FAIR

In a research study that compared how women perceived the flirtatious advances of men, researchers presented participants with a scenario: two men (one attractive and one unattractive) approach women at a party. They found that women were more likely to include the attractive male in the conversations they have with their friends, while the unattractive guy was much more likely to be told "see you later" and left in the kitchen. Second, the attractive man was more likely to secure an accurate phone number and a date. Regardless of what approach strategy was used, 55 percent of women claimed to give the attractive male an accurate phone number, nearly twice the number than gave their number to the unattractive male (28%); and women were nearly three times more likely to go on a date with the attractive male (40%) than an unattractive male (12.5%). The attractive man clearly had an advantage over the unattractive man. Also, the attractiveness of the man flirting changed the women's interpretations of the approach to communication. Women perceived that whatever an attractive male said was more inviting, playful, funny, appropriate, and less annoying compared to the same statements made by an unattractive male. Attractive men also had better luck using sexual and aggressive pickup lines than unattractive men. Unattractive men are better off using conventional, innocuous approaches to women that involve greater levels of ambiguity. Life is just not fair.

RESEARCH ON CURRENT TRENDS IN SEXUALITY AND RELATIONSHIP INITIATION: HOW WE LEARN TO COMMUNICATE ABOUT SEX

Plenty of research has been conducted on the trends of teenagers, young adults, adults, newly single adults, and even the elderly on dating, sexuality, and relationships. While individuals certainly differ in their sexual choices, research does shed light on the sexuality trends in the United States. In chapter 2, a lengthy review of how the media socialize men and women to conduct themselves in sexual relationships is presented; however, the media are not the only socialization agents involved in this process. Family, friends, peers, and relational partners help both males and females learn to communicate (or not communicate) in sexual situations and impact every level of the sexual script (cultural, interpersonal, and intrapersonal). Recall that scripts define behaviors that correspond with a culture's expectations about how sex happens: the when, where, how, why, and by whom. Adults not only provide advice to youths about sex, but model certain behaviors about sexual beliefs, communication, and practices. For example, adolescents may learn about appropriate and inappropriate behaviors by listening to adult gossip about others' sexual behaviors.

WHAT WE LEARN FROM PARENTS ABOUT SEX

People learn from parents in two main ways: first, people listen to what parents have to say about sex and relationships. Second, people observe parents in their relationships and how they talk about others' sexuality and behaviors. In general, most parents tend to talk to adolescents about sexual safely concerns, emphasizing the importance of love and commitment as a precursor for sexual activity. Parents also tend to discuss safety precautions with teenagers and how to avoid dangerous situations. Depending on how, when, and where a person grew up, advice differs, and it certainly has become more pertinent in recent decades to discuss sex with young people. This relates to an extended parenting mode where parents are responsible for their children for longer periods of time. Now, because parents are financially supporting children longer than in previous times and because children are delaying marriage, many parents play a greater, extended parenting role than ever before. Previously, parents were not overly concerned with emerging adults' sexuality because they were generally married or engaged to be married during their late adolescent years (roughly 18–22 years of age). One thing is certain: young people are not learning how to communicate about sex and relationships in meaningful ways and how to negotiate safe sex and sexually satisfying relationships that work for both partners.

WHAT WE LEARN FROM PEERS ABOUT SEX

In general, most peers talk about their own sexual experiences, emphasizing the pleasurable aspects of sex, and encourage others to engage in sexual exploration. Studies have found that peer communication is the most important factor that influences people to engage in sexual activity.[21] Friends are also the most important source for information and advice. In my study of communication about sex, people told me they were most comfortable discussing sex with their close friends, even more comfortable than with their sexual partners. This also included many married people, who said that they felt more comfortable talking to a friend about sex rather than their spouse. The downside to talking to friends is that many people do not discuss sexual health behaviors with their friends because they tend to focus on the relational aspects of their sex lives. Also, while it is fine to talk to friends about sex, this should occur in addition to speaking with the sexual partner. I think the reason why people prefer to speak to friends is that they trust and feel more comfortable with their friends.

WHAT WE LEARN IN SCHOOL ABOUT SEX

We learn very little about personal relationships or about communication in sexual relationships in secondary school. Sexual education programs vary greatly in the United States. Some school districts do not provide sexual education, some provide abstinence-only education, and some provide comprehensive safe-sex education. However, the majority of curricula fail to address and teach about interpersonal aspects of relationships and communication about sex. In a study I completed, I found that many sexual education teachers in public schools were uncomfortable teaching sexual education and were especially uncomfortable talking about sex, particularly in the classroom. This makes sense. Many of the teachers who are assigned to teach sex education are health teachers, coaches, or physical education instructors. As one woman in my study said, "I did not have any training in sex education; I didn't want training in sex education. Thank God for obesity. We are cutting our sex ed stuff in half to concentrate on weight issues, talking about eating right and exercising and stuff." Another man said, "I don't even talk about sex with my own family, my own kids, why would I be able to do it with a bunch of kids in high school? Why would I want to?"

I believe that while it is necessary to have sexual education classes that include issues of biology and reproduction and a curriculum that addresses safe sex and sexual health matters, it is also essential to have sections that cover interpersonal communication issues and communication about sex. Too often, we ignore the basic skills of communication, especially when it comes to sex. Sexual relationships are much more complicated than most people think, and having skills to talk with partners is not innate. Meaningful talk about sex does not come easy to most. Therefore adding components involving interpersonal communication perspectives to sex education curriculum would be most helpful.

BARRIERS TO CLOSE ROMANTIC RELATIONSHIPS MAY LEAD TO CASUAL SEX

In general, it seems that people are still interested in entering into long-term sexual relationships. However, there are many barriers to long-term relationships that may cause people to engage in casual sex while they are between relationships. For example, findings about the attitudes and values of college women regarding sexuality, dating, courtship, and marriage in a recent study showed that college women are still interested in long-term relationships.[22] The study reported results of in-depth interviews with a diverse group of 62 college women on 11 campuses and 20-minute telephone interviews with a nationally representative sample of 1,000 college women. For the majority of the women interviewed, marriage was a life goal, and most said they wanted to meet a spouse while at college. However, study authors found that there are several barriers in the college social scene that decrease the likelihood of women finding a mate and having a successful future marriage. They believe that relationships between college men and women today are often characterized by either too little commitment or too much, and the result is that women have few opportunities to explore the marriage worthiness of a variety of men before settling into a long-term commitment. Also, young women have a difficult time in today's world assessing the level of commitment from the men they are dating. Because of the now ambiguous relationships on campus (hooking up and friends with benefits), even the term *dating* has come to mean different things to college women. When asked to define *dating*, there was no consensus on what this term meant. Definitions of dating ranged from monogamous relationships to casual friendships. Last, the study authors found that there are not many widely recognized social norms on college campuses that define courtship, social expectations about dating, adult involvement, and guidance about relationships. While this one study by the Institute of American Values showed that women want to find a husband at college, the majority of research shows that many women do not want to be tied down in college by a boyfriend.[23] For many women, friendships are the most important kind of relationship in college.

ANOTHER BARRIER: SERIAL MONOGAMY

Many people are involved with what researchers call *serially monoga-mous* relationships. Sometime people who engage in these relationships are called *serial daters*. Serial monogamy can be described as entering into short-term sexual relationship after short-term sexual relationship.[24] It is erroneous to think that many adults are outwardly promiscuous, engaging in casual sex with multiple partners; rather, most people enter into serious, monogamous relationships. The problem is that the dura-tion of these sexual relationships is condensed, and by the end of any given year, the actual numbers of sexual partners add up to cause serious sexual health concerns. Research shows that college students take, on av-erage, three weeks to "fall in love" within their current relationship part-ner.[25] Once people consider themselves in love and in a relationship, they do not see the need for prophylactic protection (condoms) and usually rely on oral birth control for contraception. The ramifications of the idea that someone can be in love in three weeks are multiple, not only in terms of sexual health, but in terms of relational health and communi-cation about sex. People's perceptions about what it means to be in love and in a long-term relationship could become skewed. In our society, we seem to have shortened the time expectations for relationships and even sex. How many *Cosmopolitan* magazine articles, television shows, and other media encourage people to "hold out to the third or fourth date to have sex?" And moreover, how many people actually date?

Other research along these lines, by Paul Mongeau,[26] shows that in general, men have higher sexual expectations than women, particularly on dates that women initiate. However, on actual first dates, there is less sexual and communication intimacy initiated by women. Overall, men ex-pect not only more sexual contact on a first date than women, but from a communication perspective, men expect more verbal intimacy. Both men and women expect women to initiate and show more verbal intimacy than men. Of course, how well people know each other also impacts expectations on the first date. Were people strangers or good friends before the date? There are mixed results in the research regarding previ-ous relationship status and first dates. One theory is that people will be more sexually intimate (in talk and action) on the first date if they know each other because there is a higher level of comfort, and by even par-ticipating in the first date, they have decided to take their relationship to the next level. Another theory is equally compelling and states that be-cause people are already friends, there will be less intimacy on the first date because the people have more to lose, namely, the friendship itself.

So people will choose to take it slower. Different research projects support each of these theories. One outcome was clear: both men and women expected more first-date sexual intimacy when there was alcohol involved in the date.

MOVING FROM FRIENDSHIP TO ROMANCE

There has been considerable research on how people transition from friends to sexual partners.[27] One of the most important elements that differentiates a friendship from a romantic relationship—or even a friend with benefits relationship—is the mutually agreed upon definition of the relationship between the two parties.[28] That is to say, many of the same elements and levels of intimacy, emotional intensity, or sexual behavior found in a friends-with-benefits friendship and a romantic relationship are the same. One of the most important differences (if not the most important difference) comes down to how each party labels the relationship. It is clear how communication plays an essential role in the move from friends with benefits to romantic partners not only with the sexual partners, but also with how people label their relationship in the outside world. Despite that the majority of research shows that hookups rarely lead to long-term romantic relationships, there is equally compelling research that shows that friendship is an excellent place to start a romantic relationship, and if two people have already been sexually intimate, they know if there is sexual chemistry between them before they commit to a relationship. Friendship is an important foundation of a successful romantic relationship, and those who consider their spouses/partners to be close friends are generally more satisfied with their relationships than those who do not.[29] By using the "friends with benefits" label rather than calling an encounter a hookup in the first place, people in friends-with-benefits situations have already implied that they are interested in remaining friends after (and in between) sexual encounters. Recall that almost three-fourths of the college students that Mongeau surveyed had at some time been in a friends-with-benefits relationship.[30]

The often unspoken (sometimes verbally agreed upon) rules to a friends-with-benefits relationship include staying emotionally detached, specifically agreeing that neither party will fall in love or become jealous. When one person cannot help himself and falls in love, usually, the friends-with-benefits relationship ends—it either becomes a serious romantic relationship or the friendship ends. In the end, it seems that "communicating mutual love and negotiating exclusivity may be critical components of the process involved in changing a Friend with Benefits relationship into a romantic one."[31] Interestingly, in traditional romantic relationship development, the middle of the relationship (when the relationship is really escalating) is often the time of the least amount of personal disclosure and the highest period of topic avoidance because people do not want to do anything to jeopardize the relationship. This could make it difficult for some people to communicate about relationship status in a friends-with-benefits situation.

FIRST DATES

Research by Mongeau found that people go on first dates for four different reasons: to have fun, have sex, escalate the relationship, and reduce uncertainty. Specifically, men tend to report sexually oriented goals to a greater extent than do women. Women tend to report relationship oriented first-date goals (particularly, the goal of friendship) to a greater extent than do men.

What exactly is a date? As mentioned in the research by the Institute of American Values, there is no universally shared definition of a date for many people. Communication plays an important role in determining if an event is a date as well as how well the date goes. Because there is so much ambiguity in early romantic relationships, people may wonder if they went out on a date, particularly younger people. Mongeau set out to define what a date is through a large-scale research project.[32] He found that dates are dyadic in that they occur between two people rather than in a group setting. Dates had goals, meaning that dates are goal-directed events (to have fun, have sex, escalate the relationship, and reduce uncertainty). Also, dates occurred for mate selection and purposes of courtship in that both parties indicated a desire for a boyfriend/girlfriend or mate/spouse. Dates had elements that centered on the structural components of a date, specifically, a date had to be agreed upon and preplanned, it had to be initiated by a person, and a specific time had to be set.

Dates were also considered public events and included some kind of mutual activity, suggesting that dates typically occur outside of the partners' domiciles, and activity oriented indicates they revolve around some mutual activity. Interestingly, most people considered a date to be where one person paid for the other. Usually, the person initiating the date paid for the date's expenses. So using the research results by Mongeau is a good way to determine if an event was a date.

One interesting area to highlight in defining a date is that people's expectations about communication on a date are part of what makes a date a date. Most people anticipate the nature of the communication on a date. Research findings indicate that communication as a category contains general descriptions of the communication process. This means that participants describe anticipated levels of openness and appropriate amounts of self-disclosure. They anticipate polite, relaxed communication and the demonstration of social skills such as the ability to focus on the date partner. People also expect that when on a date, there will be an emotional component, that is, emotional responses partners bring to or experience on the date. These emotions range from affection (nonromantic feelings or behaviors) and attraction (physical and/or emotional attraction toward the partner) to romantic (dates have romantic overtones) behaviors.

While much of the research on dating has been done on college students, Paul Mongeau, Janet Jacobsen, and Carolyn Donnerstein found that there are some basic similarities and differences in how college students and adults view dating. College students tend to view dating as something that is dyadic and occurs in public with the goal of finding a boyfriend/girlfriend rather than a life partner. College students are more focused on physical appearance than adults. Adults tend to view dates as something that one person initiated and paid for and tend to be looking for long-term relationships. Adults are less focused on physical appearance and are more concerned with personal qualities like caring and finding someone who is a good conversationalist. Older daters are more sincere, more inhibited, and less playful than younger daters, but middle-aged daters are more physical than either younger or older daters.[33]

TABOO TOPICS IN CASUAL SEXUAL RELATIONSHIPS

Taboo topics in relational development include past relationships, other present relationships, sexual habits, sexual experiences, and the relationship status.[34] The taboo topic of relationship status is so widespread that researchers have actually studied strategies that people have to determine relationship status, other than having to communicate with the partner.[35] One of the most popular strategies was to ask a third party, such as a mutual friend, what the partner's perceptions of the relationship were or engage in relationship tests. There are different kinds of relationship tests. Public presentation tests are when a partner closely monitors how he is presented to and treated by his sexual partner's social network. Triangle tests involve fidelity checks and jealousy checks. Fidelity checks are where one person arranges a situation with a potential romantic rival and observes the partner's behavior. Jealousy checks are where one person attempts to make the person jealous and observes her reaction. Another popular alternative to direct questioning is indirect questioning, which involves hints, jokes, and an increase in touching. If all else fails, people will use direct questioning techniques as a last resort to find out about the relationship status. All these tests and strategies sound like how-to articles in *Cosmopolitan* magazine or *Men's Health*. Some of these strategies are common sense, whereas others are not so obvious. It demonstrates the lengths to which people will go to avoid the relationship talk.

It is essential to highlight that people report that they mostly feel comfortable talking about sex after they have sex; sometimes it takes long periods of time, even years, before a person feels comfortable enough to tell the truth and reveal the depth of his feelings when discussing his sexual life with his sexual partner. This has major implications for relationships. One example of a major implication is as follows: when people start having sex, patterns may become established, and it is difficult to initiate change. There are some risks—not just physical, in terms of sexually transmitted infections, but also to the relationship—involved in delaying these conversations. These risks include delaying testing for sexually transmitted infections, not discussing previous sexual relationship, and ignoring current sexual health issues. In terms of the relationship, there can also be ramifications regarding the comfort and satisfaction levels of both partners. Why is it that people can do things that they are too uncomfortable to simply talk about? This is a sexual relational phenomenon that surpasses particular cultural contexts because it is relevant in numerous cultures, people of different age groups, and different kinds of relationships.

It is the nature of relationship development that timing of self-disclosure and levels of intimacy follow their own course, and sexual activity may enter into the relationship before sufficient levels of trust and intimacy have developed for communication about that sexual activity to occur. In other words, sex and communication about sex are not necessarily the same thing and thus often do not happen at the same time. After all, many aspects of a relationship develop well before we are able or willing to communicate about them. There are real and imagined barriers preventing safer sex discussions, and more important, discussions about communication about sex in general within romantic relationships.

In a study I conducted with adults on communication about sex, I did not find any evidence that men had much information or communication about their partners' sexual satisfaction or that they were very concerned about relational maintenance as compared to what was expressed by the women. Naturally, this has implications for communication about safer sex within the relational dynamic. But what certainly did prove to be of interest to the men in the study was the issue not of whether their partners were satisfied with the sexual side of the relationship, but rather whether they themselves were people who could satisfy sexually. But men still mostly relied on nonverbal communication to determine if the women they were with were sexually satisfied.

IMPLICATIONS FOR SEX TALK

In the initiation of new relationships, communication plays a vital role. How well people communicate affects a person's ability to get a date, how well the person communicates has a significant impact on how the date goes, and how well people communicate determines if a relationship will develop and progress into something long term. Information in this chapter has highlighted the importance of mutually defining dates and relationships, particularly if one person would like a friends-with-benefits relationship to become more serious. Of particular importance in this chapter was the discussion about the timing of relationships and how this affects communication about sex.

NOTES

1. Steve Duck, "Where Do All the Kisses Go? Rapport, Positivity and Relational-Level Analyses of Interpersonal Enmeshment," *Psychological Inquiry* 1, no. 4 (1990).

2. Diane Holmberg and Samantha MacKenzie, "So Far, So Good: Scripts for Romantic Relationship Development as Predictors of Relational Well-Being," *Journal of Social and Personal Relationships* 19 (2002).

3. Timothy R. Levine, Krystyna Strzyzewski Aune, and Hee Sun Park, "Love Styles and Communication in Relationships: Partner Preferences, Initiation, and Intensification," *Communication Quarterly* 54 (2006).

4. Elaine Walster, William Walster, and Ellen Berscheid, *Equity: Theory and Research* (Boston: Allyn and Bacon, 1978), 267.

5. Steve Duck, Linda West, and L. K. Acitelli, "Sewing the Field: The Tapestry of Relationships in Life and Research," in *Handbook of Personal Relationships*, edited by Steve Duck (New York: John Wiley, 1997).

6. Helen Fisher, "Broken Hearts: The Nature and Risk of Romantic Rejection," in *Romance and Sex in Adolescence and Emerging Adulthood: Risks and Opportunities*, ed. Ann C. Crouter and Alan Booth (Mahwah, NJ: Lawrence Erlbaum Associates, 2006), 3.

7. Susan Sprecher and Pamela C. Regan, "Liking Some Things (in Some People) More Than Others: Partner Preferences in Romantic Relationships and Friendships," *Journal of Social and Personal Relationships* 19 (2002).

8. Stephanie Stewart, Heather Stinnett, and Lawrence B. Rosenfeld, "Sex Differences in Desired Characteristics of Short-Term and Long-Term Relationship Partners," *Journal of Social and Personal Relationships* 17 (2000).

9. William Graziano and Jennifer Weisho Bruce, "Attraction and the Initiation of Relationships: A Review of the Empirical Literature," in *Handbook of Relationship Initiation*, ed. Susan Sprecher, Amy Wenzel, and John Harvey (New York: Psychology Press, 2008). A review of this study is printed on p. 275.

10. In this study by Judith Langloise and her colleagues, Dr. Langloise believes that individual faces inform the perceiver of possible mutation, congenital defects, other abnormalities, and general health. The original study can be found in Judith Langloise and L. Roggman, "Attractive Faces Are Only Average," *Psychological Science*, no. 1 (1990).

11. Graziano and Bruce, "Attraction and the Initiation of Relationships."

12. Ibid.

13. Susan Sprecher and Diane Felmlee, "Insider Perspectives on Attraction," in *Handbook of Relationship Initiation*, ed. Susan Sprecher, Amy Wenzel, and John Harvey (New York: Psychology Press, 2008).

14. Graziano and Bruce, "Attraction and the Initiation of Relationships," 281.

15. Steve Duck and Susan Sprecher, "Sweet Talk: The Importance of Perceived Communication for Romantic and Friendship Attraction Experienced During a Get-Acquainted Date," *Personality and Social Psychology Bulletin* 20, no. 4 (August 1994): 391–400.

16. Walid Afifi and Alysa Lucas, "Information Seeking in the Initial Stages of Relational Development," in *Handbook of Relationship Initiation*, ed. Susan Sprecher, Amy Wenzel, and John Harvey (New York: Psychology Press, 2008), 136.

17. Ibid.

18. Levine et al., "Love Styles and Communication in Relationships."

19. Douglas T. Kenrick, Edward K. Sadalla, Gary Groth, and Melanie R. Trost, "Evolution, Traits, and the Stages of Human Courtship: Qualifying the Parental Investment Model," *Journal of Personality* 58 (1990).

20. Michael Cunningham and Anita Barbee, "Prelude to a Kiss: Nonverbal Flirting, Opening Gambits, and Other Communication Dynamics in the Initiation of Romantic Relationships," in *Handbook of Relationship Initiation*, ed. Susan Sprecher, Amy Wenzel, and John Harvey (New York: Psychology Press, 2008).

21. Allison S. Caruthers, "'Hookups' and 'Friends with Benefits': Nonrelational Sexual Encounters as Contexts of Women's Normative Sexual Development" (UMI Microform 3192595, ProQuest Information & Learning, 2006).

22. Norval Glenn and Elizabeth Marquardt, *Hooking Up, Hanging Out and Hoping for Mr. Right: College Women on Dating and Mating Today* (New York: Institute of American Values, 2001).

23. Caruthers, "'Hookups' and 'Friends with Benefits'."

24. Julie Kraut-Becher and Sevgi Aral, "Gap Length: An Important Factor in Sexually Transmitted Disease Transmission," *Sexually Transmitted Diseases* 30 (2003).

25. Seth Noar, Rick Zimmerman, and Katherine Atwood, "Safer Sex and Sexually Transmitted Infections from a Relationship Perspective," in *The Handbook of Sexuality in Close Relationships*, ed. John Harvey, Amy Wenzel, and Susan Sprecher (Mahwah, NJ: Lawrence Erlbaum Associates, 2005).

26. Paul Mongeau, Colleen Carey, and M. Williams, "First Date Initiation and Enactment: An Expectancy Violation Perspective," in *Sex Differences and Similarities in Communication*, ed. Daniel Canary and K Dindia (Hillsdale, NJ: Lawrence Erlbaum Associates, 1998). Paul Mongeau and Colleen Carey, "Who's Wooing Whom II: An Experimental Investigation of Date-Initiation and Expectancy Violation," *Western Journal of Communication* 60 (1996). Paul A. Mongeau, Janet Jacobsen, and Carolyn Donnerstein, "Defining Dates and First Date Goals: Generalizing from Undergraduates to Single Adults," *Communication Research* 34 (2007).

27. Laura Guerrero and Paul Mongeau, "On Becoming 'More Than Friends': The Transition from Friendship to Romantic Relationship," in *Handbook of Relationship Initiation*, ed. Susan Sprecher, Amy Wenzel, and John Harvey (New York: Psychology Press, 2008).

28. Ibid.

29. Ibid., 175.

30. Ibid. On p. 178, the authors cite another study done by Paul Mongeau in 2003, verifying these claims.

31. Ibid., 178.

32. Mongeau et al., "Defining Dates and First Date Goals."

33. Jeffrey Hall, Michael Cody, Grace Jackson, and Jacqueline Flesh, "Beauty and the Flirt: Attractiveness and Approaches to Relationship Initiation," in *International Communication Association* (International Communication Association, Montreal, 2008).

34. Mike Allen, Tara M. Emmers-Sommer, and Tara L. Crowell, "Couples Negotiating Safer Sex Behaviors: A Meta-Analysis of the Impact of

Conversation and Gender," in *Interpersonal Communication Research: Advances through Meta-Analysis*, ed. Raymond W. Preiss, Barbara Mae Gayle, and Nancy A. Burrell (Mahwah, NJ: Lawrence Erlbaum Associates, 2002), 265.

35. Robert A. Bell and Nancy L. Buerkel-Rothfuss, "S(He) Loves Me, S(He) Loves Me Not: Predictors of Relational Information-Seeking in Courtship and Beyond," *Communication Quarterly* 38 (1990). Leslie A. Baxter and William W. Wilmot, "Secret Tests: Social Strategies for Acquiring Information about the State of the Relationship," *Human Communication Research* 11 (1984).

CHAPTER 7

Communication about Sex in Marriage and Long-Term Relationships

"Did you see *Oprah* yesterday? The show was about sex and sex in marriages. Do you know how many married people do not have sex? She had a sex therapist on who said one of the hardest things in a relationship is talking about sex, but then they skipped over how to talk about sex and moved on to clinical stuff and how to spice up your sex life," Mary Ellen said to her friends Beth and Bridget at lunch one day.

"Oh, I feel so *Sex and the City*, eating lunch with two of my friends and talking about sex." Bridget laughed. "I didn't see the show but my sister called me about it. It's funny because I talk more about sex with you than Jerry. It is always this big thing with Jerry if I bring it up, you know? Like I am complaining about our sex life. Sometimes I just want to tell him some new information or something I heard, it's not a complaint."

"And people think women are sensitive. I don't know what it is with guys, they are so sensitive about sex. But I guess I am the only single one here so I have to worry about different things. You two are worried talking about it with your husbands, just one more reason I like being single," Beth replied. "Face it, nothing beats a good close friendship. We can talk about anything, we see each other when we want to and are completely dependable. When you need someone, you know you both can count on me."

"Yeah, I guess the grass is always greener on the other side. What really bugs me are all the jokes when you get married. Stuff like the 'shop is going to close' and what is implied is that women are the ones who are going to stop wanting sex. Like we never really liked sex, but just used to trap a guy and then once the ring is on our finger we shut up shop. For most of my friends it's the married guys who can't be bothered anymore. I wonder why that happens."

"Well, Oprah said it happens for physical and mental reasons. In part, married guys just stop asking to have sex because it's too much work."

"Too much work? I should tell you how hard single guys try to get some. It is never too much work for them. Speaking of which, I just started dating a guy. His write up on Match.com was great. He is just what I am looking for."

This is a stereotypical, fictional interaction between friends discussing sex. In this chapter, research is presented that answers many of the questions that the women asked each other and explicitly explains different ways to talk to a spouse or life partner about sex. Finding a perfect mate is not easy. In fact, relationship researchers Walid Afifi and Alysa Lucas claim that a realistic description of a personal (Internet) ad would look something like this:

> Single white female is seeking a career minded but not a workaholic male . . . should also be similar to me but different, attractive but not gorgeous, clean cut and fashion-conscious but not obsessed with looks, good conversationalist but not phony, family man but not mama's boy, independent but interdependent, committed but not smothering, loving but not possessive, sexually experienced but not overly willing, kind to others but stands up for himself, polite but not sappy, expressive but not emotional, stable and able to be fragile, fragile but able to be strong, listener, but not silent.

Initially, this is what many women are really looking for but rarely get. It is easy to imagine a similar scenario to describe a man's ideal woman, as well. However, the transition stage from casual dating relationship into a close relationship is significant. Perhaps the couple has had sex already, perhaps not, but they are definitely ready for a close relationship. What kind of sex talk is appropriate and necessary in this phase of a relationship?

INTRODUCTION

Being in a romantic relationship has many benefits that range from interpersonal satisfaction to societal approval, yet maintaining romantic relationships requires a great deal of effort and involves risks. Understanding how couples perceive and actually communicate about sex is necessary to understand the fundamental aspects and dynamics of romantic relationships. Thus, in the issues central to relational dynamics, such gender roles and expectations, self-disclosure, timing, nonverbal signs, conversation, relational development, relational maintenance, relational satisfaction, and so on are explored and connected to communication about sex. This ultimately will help people improve the quality of their romantic relationships and the ability of relational partners to have safer sex.

WHAT WE KNOW ABOUT SEX AND MARRIAGE: A REVIEW OF THE RESEARCH

As described in detail in chapter 1, marriage has significantly changed over the past 50 years in the United States. Owing to lax norms on sexual activity and the fact that people are getting married at older ages, it is likely that both men and women will enter into a marriage with a robust history of sexual experience and experimentation and have high expectations that they will find sexual pleasure in their marriage.[1] Even in marriage, with significantly decreased birthrates, contraception, and couples choosing to remain childless, for most Americans, sex is considered a recreational activity rather than one for reproduction. In fact, sex is considered so important to the success of marriage that conservative rabbis, ministers, and preachers have begun to deliver sermons about the importance of marital sex. In 2008, a trend of "sex challenges" started in many churches, where parishioners were literally challenged to have more sex. The challenges were different in range, depending on the church. For example, Relevant Church head pastor Paul Wirth, of Ybor City, Florida, challenged his congregation to have sex every day for one month. Another pastor, Ed Young of the Grapevine Church of East Texas, wanted married people in his congregation to have seven straight days of sex. Rabbi Shmuley Boteach has penned two religiously based sex books with the goal of increasing sexual pleasure in marriages, *The Kosher Sutra: Eight Sacred Secrets for Reigniting Desire and Restoring Passion for Life* and *Kosher Sex*. I use religious institutions to highlight how important sex has become to Americans because religious institutions have historically been some of the most sexually conservative institutions in America, preaching about the sins of lust. This cultural shift clearly demonstrates that ideas about marriage have changed. As sex has become further separated from reproduction, sexual activity within marriage and other close relationships, such as cohabitation, is increasingly viewed as desirable, if not mandatory, to ensure relational harmony and stability.

Sexuality in marriage is one of the most uncommon areas of study in research arenas. As noted in chapter 1, most of the research on sexuality has been driven by the increase in sexually transmitted infections, including HIV/AIDS, and focused on the negative outcomes of sex, so married relationships have been neglected in this line of research. In the United States, sexual activity is sanctioned in the marital relationship and considered morally appropriate. Due to these facts, marital sex is not viewed as a social problem or as a something likely to result in negative outcomes and therefore has not been the focus of much research in the past.[2]

In the debate about being married or single, it seems like the grass always seems greener on the other side of the fence. However, research has shown that when it comes to sex, married people are happier than single people.[3] In a landmark investigation called the National Health and Social Life Survey,[4] led by head investigator Dr. Edward Laumann, researchers found that married people expressed higher levels of emotional and physical pleasure from sex when compared to cohabitating and single sexually active people.[5] This research project is considered important in the study of communication and sexuality because it is considered to have a large number of participants. For the National Health and Social Life Survey, a sample of 3,432 Americans, aged 18–59, were interviewed, and participants completed a questionnaire with more sensitive questions about sexuality. Approximately 54 percent of the people in the sample were married, and another 7 percent were in cohabiting relationships. There is little national funding for sexuality research, and therefore samples are generally much smaller because it is so costly to conduct such research, especially research involving interviews. Due to the large number of married people in the survey, it is considered noteworthy. Results from Laumann and his group showed that 88 percent of the married individuals were either extremely or very physically pleased in their relationships. When asked about the specific feelings they experienced after having sex, a majority of the participants reported positive feelings (i.e., felt "loved" and/or "thrilled and excited"), and only a small minority reported any negative feelings (i.e., felt "anxious and worried").[6] However, in contrast to other research data on sexual frequency and satisfaction, they also found that couples who have the most frequent sex are the most sexually satisfied. The study authors conclude that Americans believe sex is essential to relational intimacy, key to personal fulfillment, and necessary to ensure a relationship lasts. Given these findings, it is surprising that an estimated 40 million Americans are in sexless marriages.[7]

Laumann and his colleagues came up with a theory of partner selection, indicating that it is in people's best interest to find one person and stay with that person and make the commitment binding by marrying that person. Their theory is called *rational choice*, which focuses on how individuals' resources and investments organize their sexual goals in modern society. If you think about it, it takes a considerable amount of time, money, and social capital to find a partner and negotiate a sexual relationship. Due to the fact that the process of securing new partners is costly, it makes better sense for individuals to satisfy their emotional and physical needs in an ongoing relationship rather than to keep switching partners. Also, while there might be the initial thrill of a new date or sexual partner, people who are in committed relationships invest in skills that enhance the emotional and physical pleasure of a particular partner. Therefore sex with a partner who knows what one likes and how to provide it is going to be more satisfying than sex with a partner who lacks such skills. Also, according to this theory, people who are in committed relationships have more incentive to invest in partner-pleasing skills if they expect a relationship to last. It makes sense that people do not find one-night stands as pleasing as sex in a committed relationship, not just for emotional reasons, but for physical reasons. Theoretically, the more committed you are to the relationship, the more willing you are to invest in partner pleasing and accommodate your partner. In terms of finding another partner, according to this theory, people are discouraged from finding alternative partners by thinking of the negative consequences of having sex with another person. It is not so much that people do not want to have sex with other people, but imagine that it is not worth the subsequent consequences.

Marriage and cohabitation both offer forms of commitment and sexual exclusivity, but because the social rules of marriage are so much more clear and universal (sexual and emotional fidelity are expected), there is a lot less negotiation necessary. In marriage, communication about sex does not necessarily have to include some of the topics that cohabitating and long-term couples need to negotiate. Research about couples who live together showed that at least one of the people had lower levels of commitment to the other and to the relationship. Also, couples who do not plan to marry show lower levels of relational satisfaction than married couples. Given the fact that married couples are more committed to each other and the relationship, it makes sense that married couples would have more of an incentive than cohabiting couples to develop "relationship-specific capital."[8] In the theory of relational choice, capital is called relationship specific because the skills learned for a particular relationship and the investment made in the relationship are not (as) valuable in other relationships. In other words, how you learn to please one partner is probably specific to that partner and is rarely transferable to another relationship. In addition, Dr. Laumann and his colleagues found that almost all of the people in long-term relationships where the couple lived together but were not married said they expected the relationship to be sexually exclusive; however, results showed that they are much less likely than married individuals to have a monogamous relationship with their partners. Based on this research, it is easy to conclude that marriage significantly increases the likelihood of a monogamous sexual relationship.

It is interesting to consider Laumanns basic premise: it is in people's best interest to marry and remain faithful to one person because married people are more emotionally and sexually satisfied that people who are not married in the face of other research that states sexual frequency declines with marriage. Many people consider sexual frequency a measure of a good marriage.

The National Survey of Families and Households included 13,000 Americans randomly selected to complete a self-administered questionnaire that included a question on the frequency of sexual intercourse. Married people reported having sex on average 6.3 times per month. Couples under the age of 24 had sex on average 11.7 times per month, and the results showed that the frequency of sex declined with each subsequent age group. The oldest age group of 75 and older reported having sex slightly less than once per month.[9] Also, duration of marriage affected frequency and desire for sex: after two years of marriage, couples reported losing interest in sex and decreased frequency of intercourse.[10] Since research shows that the frequency of sex declines with marital duration—yet Laumann found that marital sex is more satisfying to people—can we assume that it is the quality of sex rather than the quantity of sex that it is important? This is interesting, given that people also decide if their marriage is healthy, in part, on the quantity of sex that they have with their spouse. Making bold claims about research findings regarding marital sex is difficult as there are so many seemingly opposing studies.

There have been a few studies regarding the impact of communication about sex in marriages. One study included 402 married individuals who filled out a mail survey about sexual communication satisfaction, sexual satisfaction, and how the couple adjusted in the marital relationship. Results from this study showed that satisfaction with sexual communication was significant and related to improved sexual satisfaction, improved adjustment to the marriage, relationship satisfaction, cohesion and commitment to the marriage, increased expression of affection, and improved consensus in the couple. The communication of affection is directly related to an individual's happiness and marital happiness, as well. Couples that communicated affection verbally and nonverbally actually had lower levels of stress. Researchers Kory Floyd and Sarah Riforgiate studied affection and the hormonal markers of stress regulation, including cortisol, dehydroepiandrosterone-sulfate, and their ratio, and proved scientifically that the two are linked.[11] Therefore the communication of affection is seen as one of the most consequential communicative behaviors for the formation and maintenance of marriages. Another form of communication, sexual self-disclosure, has been found to improve relationship satisfaction.

SELF-DISCLOSURE IN A CLOSE RELATIONSHIP

Self-disclosure is the intentional and voluntary activity of revealing personal information, thoughts, and feelings to at least one other person. Some of these areas include private regulation and levels of informativeness and truthfulness. Privacy regulation is the level of control the people in the interaction (both the disclosee and discloser) have over the process of what is said and heard as well as who owns the information and how the information will be protected. Private information is in the hands of both people, one managing how much information will be given based on a level of trust and one who chooses whether to keep the secrets. Often people become more private and less willing to share details, especially sexual details, with their friends when a relationship becomes close. With disclosure about sex between people in close relationships, there is an expectation of more privacy and an expectation of more disclosure. Informativeness is the level of information each person chooses to disclose. In self-disclosure, people often provide incomplete sexual histories; a person may not choose to reveal sexual hangups or fantasies in a casual or close relationship. Truthfulness is more than just telling the truth or a fabrication; rather it is the level to which one reveals her true or authentic self during the casual stage of relationship initiation.

A number of interpersonal communication theories demonstrate the importance of self-disclosure in relationships. One of them is called *social penetration theory*, which says that close relationships are maintained by the gradual overlapping and exploration of mutual selves by two people in a relationship. According to this theory, close relationship growth can be predicted by and based on the number of different topics people discuss, how much time is spent talking about a specific topic, and the level of intimacy of self-disclosure. There is the slow penetration of the social identity of a person, moving from receiving and sharing surface-level information to information that is more and more personal. This is generally a linear process, and those who share too much too fast have a hard time maintaining relationships, just as those who do not share enough risk losing a person with whom they would like to be involved. Social penetration theory also recognizes that there are normal ebbs and flows and dips in relational disclosure.

Appropriate disclosure about sexual likes, dislikes, and history can be navigated using social penetration theory because the time and depth of the disclosure are very important and follow a linear path of gradually increasing disclosure as the relationship progresses. However, for many people, it is difficult to know when it is appropriate to disclose personal sexual information. Researchers know that many married people never completely fully disclose. This is acceptable because in many cases, full disclosure is not healthy for the long-term relationship either. An important aspect to social penetration theory is that relationships are viewed as entities that are continually growing and developing. A key piece in the continuation, growth, and development of sexual relationships is open communication. One problem with social penetration theory is that it was developed in the 1970s, when most relationships did develop in a linear manner; however, today, many people do not have traditional relational timing. Relationships develop at different rates; some develop quite quickly, and they are not always linear in process. Recall that most college students consider themselves in love with a partner after three weeks of dating.

Self-disclosure about sexual issues is risky at any stage in the relationship. However, it seems particularly important and risky in transitioning from a casual to close relationship. There are certain things that will always be unknown about a partner such as the other person's reaction to the disclosure and whether the person will tell anyone else about the disclosure. It is important to consider differences in what people consider private sexual information and information that is acceptable to share with friends. Conventional wisdom says that women are notorious for sharing personal information about their husbands or significant others with their friends. There have been so many television episodes that revolve around this plotline that it would be impossible to count them. It usually goes something like this: the man gets his courage up to share a sexual fantasy with his wife/girlfriend, she tells her friends, and then the friends make fun of or tease the man about his fantasy. If gossip or a third party finding out about the disclosure is a concern, it is best to clarify that you want the disclosure kept secret between the two of you. Remember, people vary on what they consider information too intimate to share.

A significant influence on the likelihood of freely disclosing sexual information is the conversational responsiveness of the participants. Reactions to the disclosure and the willingness to participate in a conversation greatly influence the success of a conversation by the disclosee. In truth, we all share a notion of a *norm of disclosure reciprocity*, which says if we disclose something, then the other person will reciprocate with a disclosure. When this does not happen, the discloser will likely experience reluctance to keep disclosing, especially if he receives warning signs that the person is not comfortable with the conversation. People do not necessarily have to have tit-for-tat disclosure exchanges, but at the very least, people need to demonstrate interest in the disclosure and support for the discloser. If people feel understood, validated and nurtured then they are still likely to say that an interaction with limited reciprocity of self disclosure was intimate.[12] In turn, the discloser has to show appropriate appreciation of the person for listening and making him feel validated. Self-disclosure about sexual needs, likes and dislikes, and even fantasies is important in married relationships. Also, starting a conversation about sex with a personal disclosure may help the other person feel more responsive to a talk, due to the norms of disclosure. It is a nice way to begin a conversation without putting the other person on the defensive.

As a final warning, it is recommended that people monitor their levels of self-disclosure carefully, especially at the beginning of a relationship. Brian Spitzberg and William Cupach, communication scholars who study stalking behaviors, believe that self-disclosure rates are an excellent measure of healthy relationships.[13] For example, stalkers' disclosures are excessive, premature, and one-sided. These are often indicators of instability. Furthermore, in stalking relationships, closeness in a relationship is found through privacy violations rather than mutual information exchanges. These signs are warning bells for everyone, so it is important to carefully monitor disclosures.

Wrapped up in the idea of comfort with communicating about sex are many relational issues besides self-disclosure: trust, commitment level of the relationship, time in the relationship, and level of intimacy. Communication scholar Sandra Petronio believes that partners in a relational system erect boundaries to maintain a balance between autonomy and vulnerability when disclosing and receiving private information from the other. So individuals in a relational system strategically regulate their communication boundaries to minimize risks and potential vulnerability.[14] Self-disclosure is a balancing act; a person has to disclose enough to establish relational intimacy, yet not too much so a person retains autonomy. This balancing act seems to be particularly relevant to the examination of disclosures about past sexual history in interpersonal relationships because it brings to light the notion of communication boundaries as a protective means for both disclosure and disclosee. In other words, this approach emphasizes the transactional nature of disclosive communication in which both partners actively exchange, negotiate, manage, and process information.

SEXUAL SATISFACTION
AND COMMUNICATION

What is the relationship between communication and sexual satisfaction? A fundamental role of communication when it comes to this is to help partners understand what each other likes. Two psychologists from Syracuse University, Daniel Purine and Michael Carey, studied what kind of sexual information is exchanged and how coordinated the couples' understandings of one another (sexually) were. For example, they wanted to see if couples shared the same sexual meanings and understanding of partner preference. "In a heterosexual couple, for example, the woman's understanding of the man's preferred sexual practices refers to the comparison between his reported preferences and her perception or estimation of his self-report. Agreement refers to the concordance between their reported preferences."[15] They found that agreement and understanding about sex were essential for high-quality marital sex.[16] If partners agree on what sexual behaviors they find pleasurable, then it is more likely that sexual interactions will be mutually acceptable and desired by both partners. This is the level of agreement about sex between couples. From a psychological standpoint, they draw attention to the fact that sex could be satisfying for a number of reasons, including the influence of other variables that might reinforce specific behaviors, rendering them "preferred" by both partners. Therefore, if a person really likes something, the other may come to like it, as well, if the other person receives positive feedback that reinforces that behavior. It has not been studied whether couples simply had a good match from the beginning of a relationship or whether satisfied couples achieved greater agreement over time, and these factors could not be determined from the study. Communication research shows that shared understanding is influenced more by communication than by agreement. So it is likely that those who communicate their sexual preferences to their partners may slowly build shared understanding over time, and eventually, both partners will find specific acts preferable and enjoyable. Because much of the burden for good sex is dependent upon the man, men are still held responsible for their own pleasure as well as the pleasure of their wives.[17] Purine and Carey recommend that marital efforts should focus on improving men's understanding of their wives' sexual preferences.

Purine and Carey also found that understanding was essential because it let one partner know how to satisfy the other. "This perspective places emphasis on specific practices that lead to the partner's physical gratification (arousal, orgasm)."[18] However, they caution that women need accurate and comprehensive self-understanding before they can share that understanding with their husbands. So it is important to metacommunicate about sexual preferences and understanding to make sure that both partners understand where each other is coming from and to be able to assess the level of agreement partners have on preferable sex acts.

In a longitudinal study of 72 newlywed couples, sexual satisfaction and changes in their sexual frequency over a six-month period of time were examined.[19] At the beginning of the study, both spouses reported their levels of sexual satisfaction and sexual frequency and completed a seven-day diary of their expectancies for sexual satisfaction. Six months later, spouses again reported their sexual satisfaction and sexual frequency. Results showed that women's sexual satisfaction was more contextually based; their reports of sexual satisfaction were based more on the actual sexual satisfaction (e.g., the sex was intimate and enjoyable), whereas men's reports of sexual satisfaction were more grounded in the physical aspects of sex such as sexual frequency. Communication is directly related to sexual satisfaction. A shared understanding of what each sexual partner considers sexually pleasing is a great place to start. It is interesting that so many people do not completely understand what their partners find pleasing, rather they inaccurately assume that they know. Also, men consider sexual frequency an important aspect of sexual satisfaction. The next section explores how to sustain sexual desire in marriage and therefore, hopefully maintain sexual frequency.

BUILDING AND MAINTAINING SEXUAL DESIRE IN MARRIAGE

The majority of research indicates that sexual desire decreases as relationship duration increases. A few research scientists have been interested in investigating ways to maintain (and increase, if necessary) a steady level of sexual desire in relationships. Sexual desire is the need or motivation to engage in sexual activities or the pleasurable anticipation of such activities in the future. Many people view sex as a chore (the dread associated with sex or talks about sex). Eliminating this view of sex would be a huge benefit to relational happiness.

Researchers Emily Impett, Amy Strachman, Eli Finkel, and Shelly Gable believe that an approach-avoidance motivational framework helps increase sexual desire over time and have completed numerous research studies to prove it.[20] Basically, people complete tasks and behave in certain ways to gain pleasure and rewards (approach goals) or to avoid punishment and unpleasantness (avoidance goals). The researchers also used the terms *approach* and *avoidance goals* to describe the reasons why people have sex. The researchers labeled people who pursued positive outcomes in their relationships and, more specifically, had sex to pursue growth, fun, and development in their relationships as those with strong approach goals. Those with weak approach goals had sex for other reasons and did not indicate they had sex for fun or for the growth or development of the relationship. They found that "people who pursue positive experiences, such as growth and development, in their relationships may view sexual activity as one way to create positive, intimate experiences with a partner. Therefore, compared with people with weak approach relationship goals, those with strong approach relationship goals may think more about sex, be more sensitive to their partners' cues, create environments that promote intimate interaction, and act more readily upon potential sexual encounters."[21] In other words, people with positive motives experience a greater number of positive events, such as desire for partners, because of a psychological process called *increased exposure*. Positive attitudes breed positive outcomes and so forth. They found that people with strong approach goals for their relationships in general may also engage in daily sexual activity for approach reasons such as pleasing a partner or enhancing intimacy in the relationship. Repeatedly engaging in sex for approach reasons, in turn, may promote greater sexual desire. For example, a man who looks at discussions about sex from an approach standpoint would want conversation to go smoothly and both people to be happy with the outcome. A man who approaches a sex talk with avoidance goals avoids conflict and wants to prevent both partners from being unhappy with the outcome. There is a big difference between the goal of both partners being happy and the goal of neither partner being unhappy.

Women who have sex for approach goals, such as to express love for their partners or because they are physically attracted to their partners, had greater levels of sexual satisfaction. Women who had sex for avoidance goals, such as to please their husbands or simply to get it over with, reported little sexual satisfaction. This means that attitude and reasons for having sex make a huge difference in a marriage. The researchers identified and tested six reasons to engage in sex: to enhance the relationship, intimacy, self-affirmation, coping, partner approval, and peer approval. They tested these six reasons against the length of the relationship, relationship satisfaction, and sexual frequency to predict daily sexual desire. People who were labeled "coping" made statements such as "I have sex to deal with the disappointments in my life." People who had sex for partner approval said, "I have sex because I don't want my partner to be angry with me." A sample peer approval statement is "I have sex just because all my friends are having sex." "I have sex to reassure myself that I am attractive" is a sample self-affirmation statement. Intimacy is more obvious; a sample statement is "I have sex to feel emotionally close to my partner."[22] They found that the approach goals enhancement and intimacy significantly predicted daily sexual desire. People who have sex for themselves or for the relationship, such as to enhance the relationship or to provide relational intimacy, desired sex every day (they may not have sex every day but indicated that they desire it). Even when the researchers tested these results against relationship, satisfaction, relationship duration, and frequency of sexual intercourse, people had much more sexual desire when they had sex for approach reasons.

When people have sex for avoidance reasons, such as to please their partners, there is much less desire to have sex. In fact, measures of avoidance of sexual goals (i.e., self-affirmation and coping) were not significantly associated with sexual desire, and the measures of avoidance of sexual goals (i.e., partner approval) were negatively associated with sexual desire. This means when people had sex just to please a partner, it actually decreased sexual desire. The bottom line is that people who are interested in pursuing growth, fun, and development in their relationships experienced a steady level of interest in sex over a six-month period of study. In addition, people oriented toward creating positive results in their relationships tend to view sex as one way to create closeness and intimacy, and their approach to sex goals may, in turn, predict greater desire during daily sexual interactions. In the end, this study showed that a positive approach to relationships in general will significantly help maintain sexual desire over time.

SKILL BUILDING: NEGOTIATING SEX

Sinikka Elliott and Debra Umberson, sociologists from the University of Texas, Austin, completed a study called "The Performance of Desire: Gender and Sexual Negotiation in Long Term Marriages." They interviewed married couples about their views of sex and how they negotiated sex in their marriages. They found that married people believe sexual intimacy in marriage is extremely important. The researchers were frequently told, "If sex is good (which, for most couples, means frequent), the marriage is okay, but if sex is bad (i.e., infrequent), the marriage is suffering. . . . Couples often experience friction over sexual frequency and describe actively working to manage their sex lives."[23] Elliott and Umberson found that in most marriages, there is a lot of conflict around sex. This main reason is that couples felt that sex was an indication or measure of the success of their marriage. Therefore, if one or both members of the couple were unsatisfied with their sex lives, then the marriage "was in bad shape."

Almost everyone in their study bought into the culturally informed idea that men need and desire more sex than women; however, this lessened the conflict around sexual issues because people thought of it as a legitimate reason for differences in sexual desire. Some even used it to justify (and forgive) affairs. However, authors stated that "wives may be less inclined to try to be sexual, and their husbands may not expect them to be sexual, because of their belief that women are naturally less sexual than men. This discourse of sexual difference stands in direct contradiction to the belief that an active sex life is an integral part of marital success. Hence, although beliefs in gender differences in sexual desire may help some couples explain away their sexual differences, forty six (74%) of the sixty two respondents report conflict over sex, especially around sexual frequency."[24]

To reduce the tension and conflict around sex, both men and women made a concerted effort to change their sexual selves: women made an effort to "want sex more often, or at a minimum be willing to have sex more often—whereas more of the husbands say that they make a conscious effort to reduce their sexual desires and focus on the quality of sex (as subjectively perceived by our respondents), rather than sexual frequency."[25] A small minority of men in the sample had less sex drive than their wives. They all reported that they were not interested in sex anymore either because of erectile dysfunction or a lack of desire. All these men were contemplating Viagra or were on Viagra but reported that they were really doing it for their wives. Most reported that even with the pill, they did not have a genuine desire to have sex. It seemed that the person in the couple (whether the man or the women) in the end made himself or herself "perform desire." "Many husbands expect wives to perform desire—whether in the form of acting more interested in sex or simply having sex more often. The husbands we interviewed say that they often wish that their wives were more interested in, and spontaneous about, sex."[26]

The researchers also found that respondents used housework to increase sexual frequency or used sex to get greater participation in housework. Many women who had paid employment outside of the home and children described sex as another form of work. Sex was like going to the office, taking care of children, and housework: basically just another chore that must be done to sustain a relationship. One man in their study reported doing most of the housework and cooking in an effort to make himself more attractive to his wife, who did not desire sex often. His strategy was that by treating her well and being affectionate, she might be more interested in sex. In summary, the authors found that

> Some married individuals, mostly wives, express a heightened awareness of the emotion work around sex that must be done to sustain their relationship, and, sometimes, resentment at having to do it. Many husbands expect their wives to be more interested in, and spontaneous about, sex. This expectation of spontaneity and authenticity increases the emotion work that wives perform around sex. Not only are they expected to have sex more often, their performance of desire should be a spontaneous, authentic response. This study also reveals the interplay and tensions between various forms of work—housework, emotion work, and paid employment—and sex in marriage. In particular, housework is central to sexual negotiation, just as it is central to how husbands and wives feel about one another.[27]

Indeed, research shows that numerous women, particularly those with young children, see sex as another chore in their relationship. Husbands' sexual expectations for women (desire, spontaneity, and authenticity) may be too much for women, given all the other demands placed on women.

It is interesting, especially given what we know about intimacy and sexuality for women, that women are often denied what they believe to be an important part of sexual and relational intimacy: conversations about the relationship and sex. Husbands may see sex talk as a waste of time or frustrating, particularly if the sex talk does not lead to sex right after the talk. If husbands believe women are pressed for time, too busy, or too tired for sex, then they cannot understand why women would have time for talk and not action. This leads to significant disagreements around the frequency of sex in marriages.

Another way people deal with conflict over sex is to joke about it. This helps diffuse the tension. It is difficult for women, who have been raised in a culture with sexual scripts that say women should not desire sex as much as men and should play hard to get, to suddenly change their worldviews once they get married. As the study authors found, it is not so easy to do.

SKILL BUILDING: COMMUNICATION APPROACHES TO AVOID AND PROMOTE

A well-known communication and marriage therapy construct is called the *demand/withdraw* pattern, whereby one spouse criticizes and nags the partner for change, while the other avoids the discussion and disengages from confrontation. According to this construct, increased demands lead to increased avoidance, which in turn leads to increased demands for engagement, with the end result being a decline in marital satisfaction. While it would be easy to think that it is typically the woman who nags and the man who withdraws, laboratory experiments that monitored actual conflict scenarios with women and men showed that it depended on the topic of discussion and the balance of power in a relationship. Both husbands and wives tended to engage in a demand pattern when they felt an issue was important to them. As far as power differences go, the person who had less power in the relationship (and often less overall relational satisfaction) tended to make more demands, while the person with more power resisted the demands and would like the relationship to remain the same. It is easy to see how conflicts around sex would take on the demand/withdraw pattern. Couples that engage in the demand/withdraw pattern have less overall satisfaction with their relationships.[28]

It is important in marriages to avoid communication that seems to be nagging or critical when talking about sex. Many of the wives in the

Elliott and Umberson study indicated that they felt nagged by their husbands to have more sex. It is not helpful if one person in the marriage feels nagged to talk about or engage in sex. Therefore it is important to address sexual issues in marriages carefully and in a positive manner. In general, open and honest communication is the best way to approach marital conflict. It is also important to stay on the topic. Often there is so much history in a marriage that it is easy to introduce old and lingering topic conflicts into a conversation about sex. Try to put yourself in the other person's shoes and realize that both people play a role in the conflict at hand. Anticipate how your responses will affect the other person and the consequences of responding in such a manner. Try to be positive, when possible, and show nonverbal and verbal signs of love and support. Whenever possible, do not reciprocate to negative responses by the other person; this will only escalate the conflict. The ultimate goal of any conflict about sex is to have two winners, not a winner and a loser. After all, it is the couple that should win when it comes to sex; when one person loses, the other can never truly win. There are more challenges for those who have an already established pattern of sexual behavior, and making changes may be difficult, particularly in introducing changes in the relationship and explaining reasons for doing so.

SKILL BUILDING: A COMMUNICATION APPROACH TO COUNSELING

It has been shown that five to six sessions of relationship education with a skills training focus reliably improve couple communication.[29] Positive effects have been shown to last up to five to seven years. This means couples tend to retain skills learned for five to seven years. Skill building includes many of the competencies that have been presented throughout the book: listening with positive nonverbal attention cues, solving conflicts where both people are satisfied, and the list goes on. Communication training can assist couples in developing a comfortable sexual vocabulary. Couples can be trained to reduce abusive verbal behaviors and use positive and direct communication. If people become anxious when they talk about sex or even in anticipating sex talk, training can also provide anxiety reduction therapy and/or cognitive-behavioral interventions. Therapy can also be helpful in identifying simple things that may improve sex such as identifying and agreeing upon the time of day or room setting that will allow one partner to feel more comfortable with sex.

One place to receive communication skills training is in counseling or therapy sessions. At what point should a married couple seek therapy for help? What can you expect in therapy for communication skills building? In a review of communication skills building programs, Tara Cornelius and Galen Alessi found that most skill building programs really focus on traditional therapy approaches. Traditional therapy provides some type of speaker-listening technique skill building. One person speaks and the other listens. This is where each person in a couple outlines his or her complaints and describes what each does not like about the other person. The partner listening is supposed to be empathetic to the other as the spouse criticizes the person. Cornelius and Alessi outline that this comes out of the Rogerian therapy model, where an individual and a therapist meet and the person complains about a third person and receives unconditional support and empathy from the therapist.

Marital relationship expert and professor of psychology John Gottman[30] believed this is inappropriate for couples therapy because couples experience an emotional gymnastics, where a partner has to listen to another complain about him and be empathetic to her, which is incongruent with his emotional and psychological state after listening to criticism. Gottman believes this may result from the immediate suppression of natural emotional responses, which is bad for communication between the couple. Gottman believes this traditional therapy approach is acceptable when the couple is complaining about a third party (a teenager, relative, or neighbor) but is destructive when it comes to the couple complaining about one another. However, the research conducted by Cornelius and Alessi found that speaker-listener techniques were somewhat successful in reducing negative communication between couples, which leads to the dissolution of relationships. Gottman recommends skill training in place of traditional therapy for most couples.

TALKING ABOUT SAFE SEX AND GETTING TESTED FOR SEXUALLY TRANSMITTED INFECTIONS IN CLOSE RELATIONSHIPS

For those involved in close relationships, there are very real challenges when it comes to talking about safe sex and taking precautions against sexually transmitted infections (STIs). Most people in close relationships, particularly marriages, believe that they are safe and in completely monogamous relationships. Yet we know from statistics about fidelity and marriage and data from the Centers for Disease Control and Prevention that both men and women cheat and bring infections home to their spouses. Another reason to talk about testing and sexual health is that numerous infections, such as HIV and herpes, can be dormant for years. Current statistics for herpes are greatly unreported because it is a dormant disease. There are numerous cases of people who misdiagnose themselves with jock itch or hemorrhoids rather than herpes because they did not think they were at risk for STIs and symptoms can appear to be similar.[31] A spouse's decision to test for STIs elicits strong emotions and doubts about fidelity. It is difficult to discuss testing and safer sex, especially in long-term couples. However, monogamy is not an effective preventative measure, and women in monogamous relationships are often provided with a false sense of safety, often deterring their use of condoms. Recall that people are more likely to use condoms in casual relationships than with regular sexual partners. Indeed, there is growing evidence that people in close relationships are putting themselves at risk for HIV and other STIs because they confuse monogamy with sexual fidelity.

The good news is that there are benefits to being in a close relationship, as individuals are in a better position to come to know if a partner is disease-free as compared to individuals in casual relationships.[32] This could be due to the fact that partners in long-term relationships have better communication about STIs. Other researchers found that people in close relationships were more likely to tell a partner if they found out they had an STI than those involved in casual encounters.[33]

A FINAL NOTE ON THE IMPORTANCE OF EVERYDAY RELATIONAL/SEXUAL COMMUNICATION

Everyday conversations are a significant and important influence on the ways in which people not only think about issues, but receive the opinions of others in their relational community and discuss the matters that are relevant to their worldviews. "Everyday discourse contains marked 'hypertext' that can be read either as an accepted part of the ordinary content of conversation or else as an item that can be 'clicked' to several further levels of meaning otherwise hidden, including a need for accounts."[34] Such hypertext can be accessed or called to account when any participant chooses to do so. One other hypertextual element of all everyday conversation, we assume, is the awareness of others' judgments and assessments that shape a person's responses and behaviors.[35] So when it comes to communication about sex, it is important to realize that the everyday communication people have with their spouses is significant in forming the relationship and the ability to relate to one another.

NOTES

1. Sinikka Elliott and Debra Umberson, "The Performance of Desire: Gender and Sexual Negotiation in Long-Term Marriages," *Journal of Marriage and Family* 70, no. 2 (2008): 393.

2. F. Scott Christopher and Susan Sprecher, "Sexuality in Marriage, Dating, and Other Relationships: A Decade Review," *Journal of Marriage and Family* 62, no. 4 (2000): 1001.

3. Linda J. Waite and Kara Joyner, "Emotional Satisfaction and Physical Pleasure in Sexual Unions: Time Horizon, Sexual Behavior, and Sexual Exclusivity," *Journal of Marriage and Family* 63, no. 1 (2001). This entire section is reviewed by Waite. See the article for details.

4. Robert T. Michael, John H. Gagnon, Edward O. Laumann, and Gina Kolata, *Sex in America: A definitive survey* (Boston: Little, Brown, 1995).

5. Waite and Joyner, "Emotional Satisfaction and Physical Pleasure in Sexual Unions." Waite and Joyner cite the original study of Laumann, which can be found at Edward Laumann, Robert Michael, and John Gagnon, "A Political History of the National Sex Survey of Adults," *Family Planning Perspectives* 26, no. 1 (1994).

6. Christopher and Sprecher, "Sexuality in Marriage, Dating, and Other Relationships," 1003.

7. Bob Berkowitz and Susan Yaeger-Berkowitz, *He's Just Not up for It Anymore: Why Men Stop Having Sex and What You Can Do about It* (New York: HarperCollins, 2007).

8. Waite and Joyner, "Emotional Satisfaction and Physical Pleasure in Sexual Unions." Waite and Joyner cite the original study, which can be found at Paula England and George Farkas, *Households, Employment, and Gender: A Social, Economic, and Demographic View* (Hawthorne, NY: Aldine, 1986).

9. Christopher and Sprecher, "Sexuality in Marriage, Dating, and Other Relationships," 1002.

10. Ibid., 1003. In a longitudinal study of newly married couples selected randomly from central Pennsylvania, researchers found that a decrease in sexual activity and interest began in the first two years of marriage.

11. Kory Floyd and Sarah Riforgiate, "Affectionate Communication Received from Spouses Predicts Stress Hormone Levels in Healthy Adults," *Communication Monographs* 75, no. 4 (2008).

12. Sandra Petronio, *Boundaries of Privacy: Dialectics of Disclosure* (Albany: State University of New York Press, 2002).

13. Spitzberg, Brian H., and William R. Cupach, eds., *The Dark Side of Close Relationships* (Mahwah, NJ: Lawrence Erlbaum Associates, 1998).

14. Sandra Petronio, *Boundaries of Privacy: Dialectics of Disclosure* (Albany: State University of New York Press, 2002).

15. Daniel M. Purnine and Michael P. Carey, "Interpersonal Communication and Sexual Adjustment: The Roles of Understanding and Agreement," *Journal of Consulting and Clinical Psychology* 65, no. 6 (1997): 1017. Helen Kaplan, *The New Sex Therapy: Active Treatment of Sexual Dysfunctions* (New York: Times Books, 1974).

16. They call it marital adjustment: adjustment to sex in marriage rather than high-quality sex.

17. Raymond C. Rosen and Sandra R. Leiblum, "A Sexual Scripting Approach to Problems of Desire," in *Sexual Desire Disorders* (New York: Guilford Press, 1988), 171. According to Drs. Rosen and Leiblum, men "are all too frequently burdened with the responsibility for arousing both themselves and their partners during a sexual encounter."

18. Purnine and Carey, "Interpersonal Communication and Sexual Adjustment," 1022.

19. James K. McNulty and Terri D. Fisher, "Gender Differences in Response to Sexual Expectancies and Changes in Sexual Frequency: A Short-Term Longitudinal Study of Sexual Satisfaction in Newly Married Couples," *Archives of Sexual Behavior* 37 (2008).

20. Emily Impett, Amy Strachman, Eli Finkel, and Shelly Gable, "Maintaining Sexual Desire in Intimate Relationships: The Importance of Approach Goals," *Journal of Personality and Social Psychology* 94, no. 5 (2008).

21. Ibid., 810.

22. Ibid., 817.

23. Elliott and Umberson, "Performance of Desire," 403.

24. Ibid., 397.

25. Ibid., 399.

26. Ibid.

27. Ibid., 403.

28. Kathleen A. Eldridge, Mia Sevier, Janice Jones, David C. Atkins, and Andrew Christensen, "Demand-Withdraw Communication in Severely Distressed, Moderately Distressed, and Nondistressed Couples: Rigidity and Polarity during Relationship and Personal Problem Discussions," *Journal of Family Psychology* 21 (2007).

29. Kim Halford, Matthew Sanders, and Brett Behrens, "Can Skills Training Prevent Relationship Problems in at-Risk Couples? Four-Year Effects of a Behavioral Relationship Education Program," *Journal of Family Psychology* 15 (2001).

30. Dr. John Gottman is an excellent source regarding couples counseling. He is world renowned for his work on marital stability and divorce prediction, involving the study of emotions, physiology, and communication. He was recently voted as one of the Top 10 Most Influential Therapists of the past quarter century by the *PsychoTherapy Networker* publication. Dr. Gottman's 30 years of breakthrough research on marriage and parenting have earned him

numerous major awards. He is a professor emeritus of psychology at the University of Washington in Seattle.

31. Walter J. Carl and Steve Duck, "How to Do Things with Relationships . . . and How Relationships Do Things with Us," in *Communication Yearbook*, ed. Pamela Kalbfleisch (Mahwah, NJ: Lawrence Erlbaum Associates, 2004).

32. Richard J. Wolitski, Bernard M. Branson, and Ann O'Leary, "'Gray Area Behaviors' and Partner Selection Strategies: Working toward a Comprehensive Approach to Reducing the Sexual Transmission of HIV," in *Beyond Condoms: Alternative Approaches to HIV Prevention* (New York: Kluwer Academic/Plenum, 2002).

33. J. Warszawski and L. Meyer, "Sex Difference in Partner Notification: Results from Three Population Based Surveys in France," *Sexually Transmitted Infections* 78, no. 1 (2002).

34. Carl and Duck, "How to Do Things with Relationships," 11–12.

35. Ibid.

CHAPTER 8

Family Communication and Sex Talk with Adolescents

Many parents are willing to discuss sexuality and sex behaviors with their adolescents; however, research has found it is often ineffective. Throughout this book, I have written about the idea of abstract and concrete communication. Abstract communication is vague and indirect, whereas concrete communication is specific and direct. In general, abstract communication is less effective than concrete communication and becomes specifically problematic in regard to family communication about sex. In fact, for many parents, when they discuss sexuality with their children, messages are often general, focusing on hypothetical situations or employing indirect strategies. Consider part of a hypothetical conversation:

> FATHER: Well, we wanted to talk to you about the birds and the bees. [*laughs*]
>
> *Teenager says nothing.*
>
> FATHER: Well, we just want you to be careful.

The father is using indirect, abstract language, and it is not effective. The attempt at humor is good, but he needs to specify exactly what he wants to talk about. There are too many topics to cover in one conversation: potential topics include physical development; interpersonal, romantic, and sexual relationships; values; and reproduction. In addition, what does *be careful* mean? Parents need to be explicit about what they would like their children to do. Does this mean be careful and not have sex, be careful when having sex, or be careful with multiple partners? And what does being careful mean when a teen is having sex? Condom use? Birth control pills? Not to get their hearts broken? Do not engage in oral sex? Consider this scenario:

FATHER: We want to talk to you about oral sex. This may be an uncomfortable topic, but it is important that we discuss it as a family.

TEENAGER: Oral sex isn't even sex. I really don't want to have this conversation with you.

FATHER: Hmmm. Thank you, Bill Clinton. So, what is sex then?

TEENAGER: You know!

FATHER: No, I don't know, because I thought oral sex was sex.

Teenager and parents have a discussion about what sex is and what oral sex is.

FATHER: Well, that is an interesting take, and you are entitled to your opinion about whether oral sex is sex. However, I think we can both agree it is a very intimate act and as such it should only be done with a lot of forethought. Also, did you know that you can get a lot of infections from oral sex? According to an infectious disease expert, Dr. Hans Schlecht, you can get human papillomavirus, gonorrhea, herpes, chlamydia, and/or, contrary to popular opinion, even HIV. In truth, it's not likely that you would get HIV, but it is a remote possibility and you should know about. Can you tell me if any of your friends are having oral sex? Do you feel any pressure to do it? If you have tried it, do you like it?

TEENAGER: Wow, Dad, that's pretty embarrassing. I don't know if I really feel comfortable telling you whether I have had oral sex. But most of my friends are doing it, and we think it's safe because you can't get pregnant doing it. It's no big deal.

FATHER: Well, it is a big deal. But I understand if you are too embarrassed to talk about it with me. Would you feel more comfortable talking to Dr. Janeway? You want me to tell you about my first experience with oral sex? It wasn't pretty . . .

They continue this conversation.

Although this hypothetical conversation is imperfect, it is realistic. The father uses concrete language and sets the stage for exactly what he wants to talk about: oral sex. Remember that you cannot cover all of what a child needs to know in one setting. The child may not know who Bill Clinton is, but the father said it anyway, more to himself. He also acknowledges his child's opinion that oral sex isn't really sex and realizes it doesn't matter that much, as long as he knows where his child is coming from and keeps the conversation going. He wants to stress that it is an important, seriously intimate act. He also asks some great questions: teens often feel more comfortable talking in the third person (teens would rather say "people like oral sex" than "I like oral sex") or talking about their friends. If a teen's friend is involved in an activity, chances are the teen is doing it as well. In the end, even if the teen is too embarrassed to talk about oral sex with the father, the father got the conversation started and opened the door to future conversations. Also, the father suggested a visit to a physician, therefore acknowledging that the teen might feel more comfortable talking about it with someone else. It is much better to have a teen talk to a physician rather than a friend about sex. Also, as indicated by research, teens would like their parents to share some of their experiences with sex, particularly their first experiences. This may not be easy to do but worth the effort and embarrassment if it has a positive impact on a teenager.

Another problematic area in parent-child communication about sex is that most topics focus on reproduction, "changes" the body might be going though, and the dangers of sex and sexuality. Many parents avoid personal issues such as the dynamics and importance of interpersonal relationships (particularly breakups), sexual pleasure, wet dreams, masturbation, and homosexuality. Sexual education programs in almost all school curricula ignore the pleasures, intimacy, logistics, and emotions related to sex, so this makes it even more important for parents to talk about these issues with their teens. Unless teens can understand and articulate what positive sexual pleasure and intimacy are, they cannot fully understand or articulate what coercive, unwanted, or detached, meaningless sex is. This is part of an important skill set to help teens avoid unwanted sexual encounters.

INTRODUCTION

Communication and interaction within families play a critical role in the development of the ability of children to create and maintain successful interpersonal relationships. The family is one of the most important socialization factors in a young person's life. Family communication patterns have been shown to significantly influence adolescents' media use; citizenship norms; consumer habits; conflict management skills; comfort communicating in a variety of situations; adjustment to college and successful separation from parents; and communication, attitudes, and behaviors about sex and alcohol use.[1] However, research shows that the majority of parents in the United States do not want to discuss sex with their children and dread conversations about sex.

Numerous family communication scholars agree that the family unit has changed significantly in the past three decades. Some major changes include that as a society, people in the United States have greatly extended the length of schooling for children, therefore their dependence on the family and, as a final result, their childhoods. In the past, many teenagers were out of the house and married in their late teens and early twenties. Now, they are in college, technical schools, or perhaps the military and are still seen as dependent on the family. Due to significant increases in the cost of living and other economic changes, children may even return to the home after college, military service, or a failed marriage, extending societal perceptions of parenthood and responsibility for children. We have smaller families in the United States compared to the past, and as a result, parents have greater discretionary income and often provide young people with goods and services that connect them to the household longer than in previous generations. The overindulgence and extended cohabilitation of teenagers means they are rarely seen as independent young adults, but rather as under the supervision, authority, and guidance of their parents. Because we have smaller families, some parents may actively seek to keep their children at home longer and avoid the empty nest syndrome. Therefore parenthood has become significantly lengthened well into the late teens and early twenties. "We have professionalized and lengthened parenthood so that parents concern themselves with every aspect of their children's lives and invade adolescent privacy. Sexual conduct, once unknown and unobserved, is covered in books, by the press, and in widely disseminated studies on teenage sexual behavior and teen culture."[2] The ignorant and uninformed parent of yesteryear is rare; the average parent today is greatly concerned by the statistics on teen pregnancy and sexually transmitted infections (STIs). Many parents do not consider it an option to talk about sexual health, as it could be a matter of life and death for their teenage children.

Other changes include cultural shifts in marriage. In our country (and others), people have begun to significantly delay marriage. In previous generations, people married in their late teens and early twenties. My mother was engaged at 19 and married and a mother by the age of 20. Her parents were not concerned about adolescent or emerging adult sexuality because it was in the confines of marriage. However, now that sex occurs for most teenagers and young adults outside of marriage, it is seen as less legitimate and necessary. Finally, previous generations were not bombarded with mediated messages of sexuality and erotica that encourage and glorify teen sex and sex in general.[3] Pepper Schwartz argues that teenagers and young adults have not changed levels in their sex drives, but rather many circumstances have changed that make it more public and less acceptable today. Her challenge to parents and society is to come to terms with teenage sexuality and accept (as difficult as it may be) teenagers and young adults as sexual beings. Data certainly support that teens are sexual creatures, with 9 out of 10 people reporting having had sexual intercourse during their teen years.

Mary Anne Fitzpatrick is a communication professor who has studied family communication for decades. She has completed numerous studies about family communication dynamics and communication between newlyweds. She believes that families have been able to adapt to change and survive, which suggests that the family unit is relatively flexible and that this flexibility is aided by how families communicate with one another. Family communication warrants separate study from other forms of communication because of the uniqueness of the family unit. However, there are similarities between romantic and familial relationships: they both contain beliefs relevant to intimacy, individuality, and affection and are influenced by external factors. The main difference is passion: passion is central to romantic relationships and not to familial relationships. Fitzpatrick and others have identified certain characteristics that determine the kind of communication families have.

The first factor is called *conversation orientation*. This is defined as "the degree to which families create a climate in which all family members are encouraged to participate in unrestrained interaction about a wide variety of topics."[4] Families that have a high level of conversational orientation communicate with one another freely, frequently, and spontaneously and do not have many time or topic limitations to conversation. In general, these families spend a significant amount of time together communicating and interacting. Family members share their individual thoughts and activities with other members of the family. Usually, when group family activities are planned, such as a vacation or an outing to the movies, these plans are discussed as a family unit and decisions are made as a family. So it is easier to set the stage for successful communication about sex within the family from a young age if other topics are discussed openly. If parents and children are accustomed to speaking with one another freely and comfortably, then the transition to sex talk is more natural. When asked about their beliefs about the role of communication in the family, families with a high conversation orientation generally believe that communication should be open and frequent between the family members and, moreover, is essential to a positive and fulfilling family life. Parents see communication with children as the most important way to educate and socialize children.

The second component to family communication is called *conformity orientation*. Conformity orientation is the degree to which family communication stresses uniformity of attitudes, values, and beliefs. Families with a high level of conformity orientation stress harmony, avoid conflicts, and have a high level of interdependence of family members. There is often respect and obedience to parents and older adults in these families. Those on the low end of the conformity orientation stress the importance of different attitudes and beliefs and the individuality of family members. Independence from the family is valued. Equality of all family members, including children, is stressed in communication. In general, families with traditional values of conformity and hierarchy tend to be those families that fit into the high conformity orientation family. Fitzpatrick believes that to assess the quality and quantity of communication in a family, one must consider both beliefs and orientations toward the family. She calls families high in both conversational orientation and conformity orientation *consensual families*. There is usually a friction between a desire to agree with one another and respect the existing hierarchy in the family and an interest in open communication and new ideas in consensual family communication. So when it comes to communication about sex, parents in consensual families are interested in their children and want to know what they think and have to say about sex, but in the end, they want to make decisions for their children. Parents often listen to their children and then spend a lot of time and energy trying to explain their points of view and decision making processes in the hope that their children will understand and accept the parents' decision and make the same decision when it comes to sexual choices.

Families that are high in conversation orientation and low in conformity are called *pluralistic* by Fitzpatrick. Here communication is open and unconstrained and involves all family members. Parents do not try to control children or their decisions; rather, family conversations occur often and opinions are evaluated on the merit of the arguments that support them. When it comes to communication about sex, in pluralistic families, parents are more willing to accept teenagers' opinions and let them participate equally in the conversation. Parents try to sway their teenagers to their points of view by using logic and reasoning and hope that their teenagers will do the right thing (whatever that may be from the family point of view).

Protective families are low in conversation orientation and high in conformity orientation. Communication is focused on obedience, and there is little room for open communication. Communication about sex in these kinds of families is limited because parental authority is seen as the most important aspect of family communication. Parents often do not see the need to explain their reasoning to their teenagers, and conversations about sex are usually limited to reproduction issues and stern "do not do it" messages.

The last combination of family dynamics is low in both conversation orientation and conformity orientation. These are called *laissez-faire families*, which means anything goes. Communication is limited to a few topics and does not occur often. Parents have a hands-off approach to parenting and believe that children should be able to make their own decisions and do not see the value in communication with children. Communication about sex in these families is usually nonexistent as parents believe teenagers should make their own decisions about their bodies and activities.

It would be helpful for each member of the family to assess the family communication style to see if each member agrees or disagrees with other members. Not everyone will view the family dynamic the same way. The family is an essential unit in helping people to become competent communicators in adolescence and into adulthood. Understanding the kind of communication in which your family engages—if they are low or high in conversation and conformity orientations—can be a helpful place to start when thinking about how to approach your teenagers about sex. If your family has a current pattern of communication, particularly one that is closed, expecting open communication about sex may be a difficult change for the family. Parents may want to start slowly with general talks about communication before jumping into talks about sex.

One of the underlying goals to communicating about sex in the family is to help socialize young adults into being competent communicators. Recall that in chapter 1, a competent communicator is described as someone who is effective in that she is able to achieve the desired goal and can meet the expected rules or expectations for the conversational context. Competent communicators possess an anticipatory mind-set, meaning that they can anticipate the implications of their actions (for both parties) and foresee any obstacle that might impede the achievement of their goals. Therefore competent communicators will adjust their goals and plans in light of situational, relational, and/or cultural circumstances.[5] Communication competence is of particular importance to the social and emotional development of teenagers. Certain communication competencies are necessary for adolescents to have, or they are likely to have fewer friendships and have been shown to have difficulty achieving intimacy in the friendships they do have. Communication competencies include verbal and nonverbal responsiveness, the ability to initiate and sustain interesting conversations, and the ability to self-disclose, offer emotional support, and manage conflict.

Deficiencies in these competencies can lead to risky behaviors and significant adjustment problems during adolescence. During adolescence, friends are seen as a principal source of emotional assistance and psychological support. Friends provide support and advice for adolescents embarking on romantic and sexual relationships. "Friends share in the vagaries of dating and romance by practicing intimacy skills, disclosing fears and uncertainties, and sorting through the subtleties of their romantic feelings—practices that may seem trivial or exhausting to adults."[6] Therefore communication competence during adolescence is essential for teens to create and maintain meaningful relationships outside the family unit. As people develop into adulthood, communication competence allows individuals to successfully access and engage peers.[7]

Family communication patterns play a significant role in teens' abilities to enact certain communication skills in friendships and romantic partnerships. Children who are raised in a pluralistic family environment with high conversation orientation are more likely to report a greater number of communication skills for both friendships and romantic partnerships than those growing up in laissez-faire or protective, high-conformity families. A research study performed regarding communication about sex within the family by Dr. Joy Koesten and colleagues confirmed that the communication competencies essential for adolescent development are more likely to be developed when the communication environment at home is one that stresses high conversation orientation and offers children a lot of opportunities for a free exchange of ideas and participation in family conversations.[8]

SEX EDUCATION AND COMMUNICATION

Most experts believe that comprehensive sex education works the best to help youths to be abstinent, provide some protection from sexual abuse, and prepare them to practice safer sex in the future.[9] This means more information about abstinence as well as reproduction, birth control, and safe-sex precautions (condom use). The least effective sexual education programs have been based on fear appeals. The common features of many fear-based curricula are as follows: (1) scare tactics, (2) contraceptive method information omissions, (3) exclusively negative consequences of sexual behavior images, (4) misinformation on medical issues, (5) sexual orientation omissions or distortions, (6) distortions of people with disabilities, (7) insensitivity to race or class, (8) religious bias, and (9) omissions in diversity of family structures.[10] Fear appeals are popular tools of persuasion when it comes to educating high school youths. Most high schools feature films and guests about automobile accidents and driving under the influence of alcohol and the dangers of drug use. These topics may be more appropriate for fear appeals: it is hard to think of a case when drinking and driving could be pleasurable and safe, at any age. However, fear appeals are not effective when it comes to sex because youths know that sex has many pleasurable aspects and it can be safe. Youths are skeptical that everything magically changes when marriage occurs, making it acceptable to have sex, whereas driving under the influence is never acceptable.

Sexual education and sexual communication are two distinct entities. In a comprehensive study of parent-child communication about sex, Jennifer Heisler outlines the difference between the two. Sexual education usually involves a teaching model of information transfer between a sender (the teacher) and a receiver (the student).[11] In this model, the sender attempts to add knowledge to receivers' frames of reference about biological reproduction, sexuality, sexual acts, and birth control. Sexual communication is the shared exchange and creation of meaning that occurs in interdependent communication encounters. From this perspective, Heisler describes family sex communication as the jointly created meanings for sex among family members. Both parents and children have an important and active role: parents influence children and children influence their parents' perspectives during these communicative exchanges.

There has been an ongoing debate among scholars about who influences teens the most when it comes to receiving information about sex, and each has data to support his or her claims. One thing is certain: every child is different, and the top three teen influences are a combination of peer, parental, and media influences. It is clear that the family, and parents, in particular, play an important part in the sexual socialization of adolescents. Both parents and children want to play lead roles in the conversations about sex. However, parents do not always make the best teachers; for example, parents may not have accurate, up-to-date information about sex or the current sexual practices of teens. Also, there is a lot of ambiguity around sex because children are unique and develop at different rates. Therefore it is impossible for a book or guide to tell parents when in a teen's development to have talks about specific topics. One thing that experts do know is that it is important to start the conversation early and keep it going in a consistent and natural manner. This is much easier said than done. It also leads people to ask, when is early? Given all these issues, it is no wonder that communicating about sex with teens can be problematic, not to mention that parents' earnest and thoughtful attempts to talk about sex may well be ignored or disdained by their children.

In a study of parents' views of sex education, only about 52 percent of parents reported feeling confident about their abilities to provide sexual education in their own homes.[12] Children's feelings about these interactions were also mixed. A majority of adolescents (61%) rated their parents as having done a "good job" with sex education.[13] Conversely, other studies found children to be frustrated with parents' approaches or critical of familial communication about sex.[14] In another study, when asked to recall sex talks with their parents, young adults stated that the talks were not positive or negative, mostly neutral.[15] Students viewed parents as doing a satisfactory job passing on information from a sex education standpoint and thought the information was very accurate. However, students rated the quality of communication with parents as rather low and indicated that they wanted more communication about sex with parents. When asked what they wanted from their parents in terms of sex talk, young adults stated they had a desire for parents to display a more positive attitude about sexuality. Parents of the young adults said they wished they had talked more about prevention and abstinence with their kids. It is obvious that parents and children have significant differences in how they perceive sex. Young adults said they felt they could have benefited from hearing about their parents' experiences, if the parents had been willing to share them. Overall, most young adult participants wanted to be more open with parents, hearing about parents' difficulties and being able to share their own experiences. Sons and daughters seemed to perceive their parents as sexual beings; that parents played multiple roles, including mom, dad, lover, and friend; and desired input from parents on these issues. Parents, on the other hand, had difficulty coming to terms with their children as sexual beings. Parents said that they wanted more open communication with their children and yet were uncomfortable with the idea of engaging in open dialogues about sex with their children.

ADOLESCENT SEX AND LOVE

While it is easy for adults to dismiss teen love or puppy love as inconsequential because adults know that puppy love is short-lived, love plays a significant role in the life of the adolescent. Dr. Helen Fisher suggests that there are numerous personal and social benefits to teen passion, romance, and sex. These benefits include "exhilarating joy, increased energy and optimism, feelings of intimacy, self-esteem, inclusion in health-giving social groups, exercise, social and personal support and crucial practice in the skills of building long term partnerships skills they will need to make the most important social contract of their reproductive lives."[16] Love and sexual experimentation are important rites of passage for young adults in the United States. In fact, adolescents consider being in a romantic relationship a central part of belonging and attaining higher levels of status in peer groups. For many teens, there is a direct link between peer status and being in a romantic relationship. Peer networks support romances and even connections to new peers/friends through the romantic relationship. Peer networks are extensively involved in the adolescent dating culture. It would be easy to imagine the depth and breadth of communication (and analysis) between friends at the beginning of a romantic relationship in the teenager's circle of friends.

We know that adolescents tell stories to negotiate and solve romantic dilemmas. During the storytelling process, the meanings of words and actions are deliberated; dilemmas arise over these meanings, many of which reveal contradictory positions that must be managed during the conversation. In an analysis of the romantic stories of young adults, researchers found that of the romantic stories that were told between friends, 80 percent focused on romantic problems, and most of the talk was problem talk and problem solving.[17] Around half of the stories in the study revolved around relationship instability. Other problems that occurred in the stories included problems of asymmetry of interest (21%), infidelity (11%), and interference from others (9%). Stories about relationship instability emphasized the ambiguous and unpredictable nature of relationships, often because of something chronic such as personality differences, communication failures, and feelings of being controlled or stifled or incompatible values or lifestyles.[18] Peers have an enormous impact on helping friends sort out sexual relationships and, in the process, make sexual decisions.

It is difficult to conduct research about adolescent sexual behaviors for many reasons—some obvious and others not so obvious. The problems with getting adults to truthfully answer questions about their sexuality are multiplied when it comes to teen populations. Often parental consent to participate in research is necessary, and even if the surveys are anonymous, teens may be afraid to admit behaviors. But on a larger level, teen culture is constantly changing and adapting and so diverse that it is only possible to capture snapshots of the sexual culture, and those are difficult to obtain. One researcher claims that studying adolescent sexual behavior is like trying to chase a greased pig.[19] However, researchers have had success in recent years gaining some insight into how teens communicate about sex. Findings indicate that adolescent sexual relationships are significantly hampered by a lack of communication between sexual partners. For many teens, sex talk is difficult and uncomfortable; however, it is of the utmost importance for health and well-being of sexually active youth. We know that adolescents who have positive attitudes toward discussing safe sex and are able to engage in contraceptive-specific sexual communication, such as discussing condoms or STIs, are more likely to use contraception. However, sexual communication should not be restricted to discussions of contraception or infections; rather, sexual communication should include discussions of a wide variety of topics such as sexual histories, sexual likes and dislikes, or sexual fantasies. Teens who can discuss these sensitive issues with their partners are much more likely to feel comfortable in their sexual relationships and are therefore more likely to have safe sex and be able to control their sexual boundaries.

Researchers Laura Widman, Deborah Welsh, James McNulty, and Katherine Little from the Department of Psychology, University of

Tennessee, Knoxville, conducted a study with 209 couples dating a minimum of four weeks who participated in the Study of Tennessee Adolescent Romantic Relationships.[20] Seventy-three adolescent dating couples (ages 14–21 years) who had sexual intercourse completed a sexual communication questionnaire. This was an interesting study because data from both partners in the sexual relationship were collected. This allowed the researchers to gain a more complete snapshot of the sexual relationship and to be able to compare stories for accuracy. Many sexually active adolescents in the study did not feel comfortable discussing sex with their partners. The researchers found that relationship length, satisfaction, and commitment impacted the quality and quantity of communication about sex in teen relationships. Highly committed adolescents reported greater sexual communication. Those adolescents who were more open sexual communicators were more likely to report using contraception, and this association persisted even after contraception communication was considered. As contraceptive use requires some planning (e.g., purchasing condoms, taking oral contraceptives in advance), it is likely that contraceptive communication preceding intercourse allows adolescents to be more prepared for sexual interactions when they occur. This directly relates to setting boundaries before the sexual act occurs and demonstrates the importance of setting boundaries prior to sexual encounters. The level of trust required to share one's feelings about sexual practices and fantasies may foster a sense of intimacy and investment in couples that allows them to commit to healthy sexual practices. The researchers also found that both male and female adolescents who were more satisfied with their romantic relationships were more open in discussing sexual topics with their romantic partners and that this association led to increased contraceptive use. They speculated that this may be due to the fact that the intimacy fostered by disclosure of sensitive sexual information is a salient bonding experience that contributed to the development of relationship satisfaction. Alternatively, it is also possible that good sexual communication improves sexual satisfaction, which in turn enhances relationship satisfaction.

Some of the less positive findings had to do with girls who *self-silence*, which is when girls tend to silence their own wishes or desires in the context of their relationships. For example, girls agreed to the statement "I think it's better to keep my feelings to myself when they conflict with my partner's" were coded as self-silencers. Based on reports of condom and birth control use in the survey, girls, but not boys, who used more self-silencing talk reported lower sexual communication and reduced contraceptive use. Psychologists believe that sexual communication is difficult for adolescents, in part because they fear their partners will react negatively to these discussions. Therefore it is not surprising that teens who avoid conflict through self-silencing are bad at communicating about sex. Furthermore, girls who self-silence are usually more likely to conform to traditional gender roles that women should be less assertive than men in sexual situations.

In a research project designed to understand how adolescents negotiate romance, sex, and love in the face of sexual disease risk, adolescents were asked to explain their worldviews on permissiveness, double standards, sexual control, and romance and how these conceptions play into their sexual decision making.[21] For the young people in this study, the perception of a committed relationship seemed to somehow grant permission for unsafe sex. Young women believed this more than men, and when the partner was a person who girls knew well, loved, and trusted, they felt it was less necessary to use condoms. Adding to this problem is the fact that women are more worried about their reputation and therefore were more likely to judge casual sexual encounters as something more meaningful and long term than men and therefore to be low risk. These are some reasons why young women do not consistently use condoms.

TEENS TALKING ABOUT CONDOMS

Teens aged 16–19 years were asked why they were reluctant to talk about contraception with lovers.[22] The hardest part for the teens was actually initiating discussions of contraception. Teens feared that if they brought up the topic of contraception, then they would not only have to admit the intention to have intercourse, but they believed there was a negative connotation between condom use and disease prevention. In other words, if a teen were to bring up condoms, the sexual partner might think the teen was dirty or diseased. There was also a perception that there would be an even more negative reaction if the partner already has a reputation of being sexually experienced. Teens also feared that their reputation would be harmed if they even brought up the topic of condoms. Sex talk could also force the dreaded "relationship talk"—and instigate a talk about whether the sexual relationship was going to be long term and birth control pills should be considered.

The reality is that most teens welcome talks with their parents about contraception and condoms. Studies show that there are very few negative responses to talks about sex, and parental fears and concerns about broaching the subject are largely unfounded. The fact is that in this study, when teens talked about condom use, condoms were used in about 80 percent of the sexual experiences, and when no talk occurred, condoms were used only 44 percent of the time—a huge difference. It is easy to understand why teens feel uncomfortable admitting to a desire for sex because teens don't want to be perceived as being pushy, too forward, or focused on sex only. Interestingly, more boys than girls were afraid of admitting to wanting sex, precisely for the reasons noted earlier. When talking to boys, it is important to help them negotiate condom use so they can talk about condom use without sounding too pushy or that they are only with a girl for sex and alleviate some of their fears. For example, assisting boys in constructing scripts may help. Boys could say something such as "I am talking about condoms because I care about you. We don't have to have sex. I will really like you whether or not we do it. But if we do it, let's use condoms." This is especially important because a lot of girls wait for boys to take the lead in condom use.

The partner's reputation was a significant factor as well in terms of likelihood of discussing and using condoms. Teens who were involved with someone popular and who had a high status among friends found it even more difficult to talk about contraception. One teen in the study said, "I was thinking about it [talking about contraception], I was laid there and I thought God, cause he's quite cool, cause I was younger . . . I saw him as a cool character you know what I mean. . . . I thought of saying have you got a condom . . . I thought I can't say that it's un-cool . . . I was so scared of his reaction."[23] Given the fact that so many teen girls date older guys, it is important for parents to be aware of the additional pressures and fears that girls will face with popular older guys.

PARENTAL INVOLVEMENT IN COMMUNICATION ABOUT SEX: YOU ARE DOING BETTER THAN YOUR PARENTS DID, BUT IS IT GOOD ENOUGH?

Teens report that they receive more information about sex from informal sources, such as peers (especially same-sex friends), than from any other source.[24] Common sources include dating partners, opposite-sex friends, the media, and reading on one's own (including the Internet).

Formal sources, such as parents and teachers, provide only a small amount of information, and fathers were reported to give far less information than mothers. One possible reason for this is that most communication about sex occurs among peers, and therefore peers are the greatest source of information, as well. In fact, same-sex friends and dating partners are the two types of people with whom adolescents communicate the most about sex. Some studies show that students say that they rarely, if ever, discussed sex with their parents, and conversations that did occur tended to be with same-sex parents.

Consider Jennifer Heisler's comprehensive study of parent-child communication about sex. She asked both college students and their parents to recall their conversations about sex and safe sex and found that students' and parents' memories of talks about sex were really different. Parents remembered (or thought) that they talked a lot more about sex than teens recalled. The differences were not just in frequency, but in the quantity of topics. Students remembered discussing fewer topics with both mothers and fathers in comparison to parental recollections. The biggest differences were between mothers' and children's recollections of sex talk. These differences may just be in perceptions as to what is personally salient to individuals. The fact that mothers saw these past discussions very differently than their teens could be because mothers' recollections reflect cultural standards for good mothering behaviors because social rules say that mothers should talk about sex with their kids. Most women still have the role of family caretaker, and as such, mothers might feel a greater responsibility to protect other family members and want to show others (e.g., within the survey) that they had managed and cared for their children through talks about sexuality and relationships.

Almost all the participants recalled that mothers talked about sexuality more often than fathers and believed that mothers were more comfortable and open than fathers. Mothers also indicated greater comfort with these topics than did fathers. "Culturally this is similar to other research findings that show mothers remained the 'in-house' expert on relationships. Although sons ranked fathers [as a] significantly higher source of information than daughters, sons still recalled a preference for mothers over fathers. Because discussions about sexuality provide information for young adults beyond factual knowledge (e.g., who talks, who does not, who is warned, who is encouraged), fathers' silence may continue to perpetuate socialized gender roles concerning sex."[25]

Both parents and students agreed that the focus of parental sex talks were on negative consequences of sex such as STIs, unplanned pregnancies (even for boys), and morality. This could be that parents thought these topics would lead to abstinence more than other topics. Not surprisingly, both parents and students also agreed that homosexuality, infidelity, the timing of sexual initiation, and peer pressure were the least discussed topics—which are considered taboo topics by many families. Maybe parents did not think that these topics were important, especially those topics that involved infidelity and peer pressure. Clearly these taboo topics are not fully understood by parents, and even some students did not feel comfortable addressing the pressures they were facing from boyfriends or girlfriends, concerns about infidelity, or their sexuality identity with parents and therefore avoided the topics if parents did bring them up. Interestingly, overall, mothers, fathers, and children all reported that they were moderately satisfied with their family communication about sex. Dr. Heisler speculates that parental satisfaction with overall communication might be due to evaluation based on the sexual education model of *information transfer*—giving children the basics of the birds and the bees. In other words, in terms of sex education, parents may feel responsible for providing information about STIs, pregnancy, and the menstrual cycle.

In Allison Caruthers's study on college women who hook up, the majority of participants reported difficulty in having serious conversations about sex, especially with their parents. Most women stated that their parents gave them basic information about procreation but nothing about how to act in a sexual relationship or how to communicate feelings and needs with partners.

As demonstrated by these research findings, another problematic area in parent-child communication about sex is that most topics focus on reproduction, "changes" the body might be going though, and the dangers of sex and sexuality. As previously mentioned, many parents avoid personal issues, and sexual education programs in almost all school curricula ignore emotions that occur from sexual experiences, including pleasure. This makes it even more essential for parents to talk to their children about these ignored issues.

SUPPORTING THE TEEN AFTER A BREAKUP: REFLECTING ON SEXUAL EXPERIENCES

One of the most important times parents can be there for their children is after a breakup. After having received many of the benefits of love, losing both the benefits of love and the boyfriend may seem overwhelming to many teens. It would be easy for parents and other adults to trivialize breakups, especially because adults know that breaking up is normal for teenagers and the pain is relatively short-lived. But the pain that results from rejection is very real for teens and warrants parental attention. This is an important part of communication about sex. Some researchers argue that breakups and relationships are particularly difficult for teens because of brain activation and biology that make teenagers lack impulse control and emotionally different from adults due to hormone changes. Others consider it a factor of social construction in that teenagers have not learned how to control their emotions or benefit from previous experiences to help them make sense of the world around them. Whatever the reason, breaking up is significant and devastating to teenagers.

Pepper Schwartz would go further to argue that teens are actually quite like adults if you really look at the similarities. For example, teens are likely to have more dating partners, and therefore society considers sexual intercourse among teenagers sporadic. However, Schwartz believes that if we were to compare condom use and contraception among adults who have the same irregular sexual patterns as adolescents, we would find more similarities than differences.[26] Indeed, some of the significant differences between teen breakups and adult breakups are due to the fact that teen breakups occur in a fishbowl. Teenagers are more likely to lose social status and friendships as a result of a breakup compared to adults. Because teens are in high school, there is likely to be much gossip surrounding the breakup, affording the rejected person little privacy. Not only are people talking about a person's loss, but doing so daily, rarely tiring of the subject. The rejected teen has little chance to avoid his ex and probably even has to see her with a new person. This would be tough for an adult, but fortunately, most adults are able to completely separate after a breakup, whereas most teenagers are not so lucky. For most teens, the teen breakup is "experienced in a group context; there is one voice to judge romantic and sexual dramas and decide who is right or wrong and indeed every detail of the action. When young people complain to their parents, saying 'everyone thinks' they are not as misguided as their parents might think—remember this is a group that walks in lock-step to music, clothes, dance, and idols."[27]

After a breakup is an excellent time to talk to adolescents about sex, romance, love, and survival. Parents can help teens reflect on their decisions, their sexual experiences and consequences, and whether they engaged in appropriate levels of intimacy. Parents can ask their children if there were any ramifications to their reputation and, in general, talk about the nature of interpersonal relationships.

ADOLESCENTS' SEXUAL DECISION-MAKING PROCESSES, COMMUNICATION COMPETENCE, AND RESISTANCE STRATEGIES

There are implicit and explicit sexual offers that your child will face. Explicit offers are direct requests from the boyfriend or girlfriend: "Do you want to have sex?" "If you love me, you should do it with me." But remember that there are also implicit pressures to have sex, as well; these are indirect pressures. Perhaps all their friends are doing it or they are at parties and people are doing it. Sex is something people cannot avoid; the media propagate sexual activity constantly. To avoid unwanted sex, teens can use a direct no response, they can offer an excuse, or they can avoid the person or friends by whom they are feeling pressured.

Pediatricians at the University of California, Tricia Michels and Bonnie Halpern-Felsher, along with other colleagues interviewed ninth-grade adolescents to find out how they perceive the initiation of part-nered sexual experiences, including anticipated future sexual activity. They found that adolescent sexual decision making is based on rela-tionship value and personal characteristics, social and health risks and benefits, explicit decisions regarding boundaries, and an active evalua-tion of sexual decisions when presented with opportunities to have sex. The ninth graders engaged in a variety of sexual behaviors that ranged from vaginal sex, deciding to engage in other sexual behavior, opting not to engage in sex when faced with the opportunity, or avoiding oppor-tunities altogether. Their analysis revealed that the decision-making process remained relatively stable across sexual behaviors; that is, they all used the same decision-making processes. Boys in their study empha-sized the importance of a partner's reputation and past sexual history. More often, boys were willing and able to engage in sexual intercourse if a girl had a reputation as being experienced. Boys and girls consid-ered personal attributes of readiness and feared disrupting their lives with the potential negative outcomes of sexual activity. Both boys and girls evaluated their abilities to care for a child with their current part-ner should that be the outcome of a sexual encounter. At the same time, boys and girls shared positive views of sexuality as part of their normal development. The main reason they had sex was for sexual pleasure and relationship enhancement.

Another interesting finding in this study particularly relevant to sex talk was the confirmation of the importance of boundary communication; that is, many of the adolescents described constructing boundaries first, then communicating those boundaries to potential sexual partners. Michels and Halpern-Felsher reported that some girls discussed limits before the sexual event. For example, one sexually experienced girl said, "I told him I'm not ready to have . . . actual sex; fooling around is OK, but actually having sex, I don't want to do that." She set a boundary: no sex. Teens who set boundaries and discussed them before fooling around reported they were much more comfortable and successful talking about sex and saying no compared to those who negotiated the boundary in the moment. In the moment, negotiation was not always bad, as another ninth grader said: "There was a point where both pants were off at the same time. It was up in the air, like you could tell it wasn't set, but you could just tell, and I just shook my head and said, 'No, not now.' And he said, 'OK, I'm fine with that.' I said, 'Good, because if you weren't, it'd be a problem.'"[28]

Some of the nonexperienced girls had communicated their boundaries clearly to their partners and successfully avoided sexual encounters, but a few failed to verbally communicate their boundaries, assuming incorrectly that their partners shared their feelings. For example, one girl described her encounter of having the opportunity to have sex but choosing not to as "really awkward. . . . I almost broke up with him for that, because I didn't feel like we had the same mind-set." She had not discussed her boundaries in advance because "I didn't think that he would ever want to." Another young woman who failed to communicate her boundaries with her partner before the experience described much more discomfort during the sexual event: "We were just kissing and then all of a sudden he just whipped it out. And I was like, Whoa! I hope he doesn't think I'm going to do anything with him. . . . I didn't think he would do that to me."

The experienced boys and those with opportunities to have sex communicated boundaries to their partners both directly ("I told her straight out") and indirectly ("I made up an excuse"). One boy experienced with oral sex explained his communication about boundaries: "We both made it clear that we both wanted something to happen, just by little gestures or comments we made. . . . We [also] made [the limit] clear to each other. You can tell, you know, just like a presence: that's as good as it's going to get for today." The adolescents often described their sexual experiences as spontaneous—as one experienced girl said, "It just happened"—but most indicated communication and decision making beforehand: "We [had talked about] when our first time was going to be, the surroundings, the environment, how it was going to be" (experienced boy). Ultimately, the goal of boundary communication is for the two partners to find shared boundaries about sexual limits and safety behaviors.

Dr. Claude Miller, an expert on sexual communication and adolescents, offers some talking points for sex talk with teens.[29] First, Miller believes that parents should know a bit about psychology when it comes to speaking with teens. Of particular importance is *psychological reactant theory*, which is the notion that if you tell someone what to do, she will have a tendency to do the opposite. Miller believes that when a parent provides any sort of persuasive message telling a teen what to do, it could have the opposite reaction and encourage the teen to do the opposite of what the parent wants the teen to do. Research has shown that teens are particularly susceptible to psychological reactant theory, especially when it comes to messages about drugs and sex. Often parents craft messages that cause more harm than good, and parents can actually cause children to try to restore the threatened freedom that a direct style of communication creates. Miller offered this example: if you tell a child he can't smoke, he anticipates that he has a freedom to smoke and that freedom is threatened, so he goes out and smokes to restore his freedom, even though he may have had no plan to smoke in the first place.

With psychological reactant theory in mind, Miller believes the best way to approach persuasive messages with teens is to use implicit language rather concrete language when it comes to advice. Parents should avoid commands or direct suggestions and controlling language. It is best to use questions such as "can we consider this?" and soft statements such as "you might want to think of this when you are making your decision." This is what psychologists call *autonomy-forming language* because it allows the teen to engage in the conversation without feeling defensive. Also, parents should not stopping talking with their older children once they leave the house, especially if they are in college. During this time, called *emerging adulthood*, young adults have a lot of freedoms that they think adults should have but are not used to. Plus they differ from adolescents and adults in that they have a lot more freedom because they are not living under the direct control of parents and do not have the responsibility of being in the workforce with careers and families. Given these combinations, emerging adults are prone to take many more sexual and health risks.

TALKING TO TEENS ABOUT SEX

Parents should consider the following approaches:

- Don't use controlling, explicit language when it comes to giving advice. You want your child to feel as though she came up with an idea or made a decision.

- Do use concrete language when providing sexual health information or topics you would like to discuss with your teen. Specific messages are as important as the way in which the messages are communicated. Adolescents say that they want their parents to be open and comfortable. They do want sexual information from their parents—they might not act like it, but they really do.

- If you do use explicit language for advice giving, let teens know exactly what you want, but then give them a method to restore their freedom. One thing teens could do is ignore you, put you down, and this would cause you to lose your credibility in the future. Emphasize that they have a choice. You get your message across, "Don't have sex," but then say, "But it is really your choice, you have to decide." This way, you do restore their freedom; it's not so much that emerging adults want to participate in risky behaviors, but that they want the freedom to choose to do it. Parents could say, "You could do it if you wanted to, your friend does it, and you can if you want to." Remember that teens want to think that they are in control and self-determined. In the end, it is true that parents cannot really control their children, but they can give them the tools to make wise decisions. Mostly important, don't threaten their freedom or their perception of freedom.

- Make sure both mothers and fathers get involved with sex education.

- Make sure you start early. Experts usually recommend that parents talk about sex from the ages of 13–19 years. However, parents can make sexual communication a process, for example, by talking to younger children about how to dress modestly or respect the opposite sex.

- Simply letting your child know you are open and willing to talk is helpful, and parents should be open to talk if they are approached.

- Be clear about expectations for behaviors and be honest and clear about your own views and beliefs.

- Perhaps the most difficult thing for parents to do is discuss sexuality in a positive manner and accept the possibility of sexual activity by discussing birth control and accommodating children as equals in communicative interactions. Accepting that your children play additional roles, such as "lover" or "friend," can go a long way.

- Encourage your child to set boundaries with their significant others and talk about sex in their relationships.

- Offer an alternative person to provide accurate health information, such as a physician or nurse, if a teen indicates that he is too uncomfortable to talk to a parent about sexual health. Speaking with a health professional is much better for teens than getting information from friends.

- While it is clearly acknowledged (and with good reason) that for some parents, talking about sex with children is purposely avoided out of fear of encouraging promiscuity or sexual exploration, it is best to talk about it to prevent serious consequences.

- Know your terms and make sure you share meanings about sexual terms with your teen.

Some statistics about teenage sexual behaviors follow:

- More than one-third of new HIV infections in the United States are among persons ages 13–29.[30]

- It is estimated that approximately 40 percent of male adolescents and 30 percent of female adolescents have had vaginal intercourse by the ninth grade. Prior to vaginal intercourse, 30 percent of adolescents report heterosexual masturbation with a partner, 10 percent have had heterosexual oral sex, and 1 percent have had heterosexual anal sex.[31]

- Anal sex among teens is on the rise. Researchers cite a number of reasons anal sex is becoming more common, including fear of pregnancy, the desire to preserve virginity, and the popularity of anal sex in pornography. A 2005 study based on data from the National Longitudinal Study of Adolescent Health found that while teens who took virginity pledges had sex later and had fewer partners overall, they were more likely to have oral and anal sex and less likely to use condoms. Rates of STIs among pledging and nonpledging teens were similar.

- None of the ninth graders in the Michels study considered kissing, "making out," or "touching" to be sexual activities.[32]

- One study revealed almost 30 percent of adolescent couples failed to use contraception the first time they had sex and nearly half of these couples did not use contraception every time they had sex.[33] These statistics are discouraging given the prevalence of AIDS, STIs, and unintended pregnancies among sexually active youth.

- In a 2008 study of 1,348 at-risk youths ages 15–21 in three U.S. cities, Celia Lescano of Bradley Hasbro Children's Research Center in Rhode Island and colleagues found that 16 percent of participants reported recent heterosexual anal intercourse. "Given the subject matter, it is likely that the numbers reported may actually be an underestimate of the prevalence of these behaviors," Lescano said. "There is no doubt that teens lack information about STDs and the safety of different behaviors, and they are engaging in more sexual experimentation." Even though the topic of anal sex is often considered taboo, Lescano urges "open discussion" of its consequences in doctor's offices, within sexual relationships, and with parents.[34]

- Longitudinal data from over 10,000 13- to 16-year-olds who participated in randomized trials of school sex education in the United Kingdom were tested to measure the amount of pressure students felt to engage in first intercourse and if they regretted it, pressure and enjoyment at most recent intercourse, and general relationship quality. Of the 42 percent of youths who reported having had sex by follow-up, most assessed their first and most recent sexual relationships positively. Greater proportions of females than males felt pressure at first sexual intercourse (19% vs. 10%), regretted their first time (38% vs. 20%), and did not enjoy their most recent sex (12% vs. 5%). The younger people were when they first had sex, the more they regretted it. Negative sexual experiences were associated with less control (e.g., feeling pressure, being drunk or stoned, or not planning sex) and with less intimacy (e.g., sex with a casual partner or less frequent sex). Interestingly, those who felt pressure at first sex were most likely to be female and reported poor communication with parents and regular drug use. Also, having had oral sex, greater frequency of sex in the last 12 months, and having a boyfriend or girlfriend rather than a casual partner were associated with a lack of enjoyment. Anticipated ease of communicating with one's partner remained associated with enjoyment of physical contact and became a predictor of enjoyment of time spent with a partner; quality of relationships with boyfriends or girlfriends was positively associated with physical and emotional intimacy.[35]

NOTES

1. Joy Koesten, "Family Communication Patterns, Sex of Subject, and Communication Competence," *Communication Monographs* 71 (2004).

2. Pepper Schwartz, Ann C. Crouter, and Alan Booth, "What Elicits Romance, Passion, and Attachment, and How Do They Affect Our Lives throughout the Life Cycle?" in *Romance and Sex in Adolescence and Emerging Adulthood: Risks and Opportunities*, ed. Ann C. Crouter and Alan Booth (Mahwah, NJ: Lawrence Erlbaum Associates, 2006), 55.

3. For a complete discussion of changes in families, please see Philip Blumstein and Pepper Schwartz, *American Couples: Money, Work, Sex* (New York: Morrow, 1983).

4. Ascan F. Koerner and Mary Anne Fitzpatrick, "Toward a Theory of Family Communication," *Communication Theory* 12 (2002): 85.

5. Koesten, "Family Communication Patterns."

6. Neill Korobov and Avril Thorne, "How Late-Adolescent Friends Share Stories about Relationships: The Importance of Mitigating the Seriousness of Romantic Problems," *Journal of Social and Personal Relationships* 24 (2007): 972.

7. For a complete review of the information presented in this paragraph, please see Koesten, "Family Communication Patterns."

8. See Koesten, "Family Communication Patterns," for a complete review of this subject.

9. K. Haglund, "Recommendations for Sexuality Education for Early Adolescents," *Journal of Obstetric, Gynecologic, and Neonatal Nursing* 35, no. 3 (2006).

10. L. M. Kantor, "Scared Chaste? Fear-Based Educational Curricula," *SIECUS Report* 21, no. 2 (1993).

11. Jennifer M. Heisler, "Family Communication about Sex: Parents and College-Aged Offspring Recall Discussion Topics, Satisfaction, and Parental Involvement," *Journal of Family Communication* 5 (2005).

12. K. J. Welshimer and S. E. Harris, "A Survey of Rural Parents' Attitudes toward Sexuality Education," *Journal of School Health* 64, no. 9 (1994).

13. Alexander McKay and Philippa Holowaty, "Sexual Health Education: A Study of Adolescents' Opinions, Self-Perceived Needs, and Current and Preferred Sources of Information," *Canadian Journal of Human Sexuality* 6, no. 1 (1997).

14. Christine L. Young Pistella and Frank A. Bonati, "Adolescent Women's Recommendations for Enhanced Parent-Adolescent Communication about Sexual Behavior," *Child and Adolescent Social Work Journal* 16 (1999).

15. Heisler, "Family Communication about Sex," 306–7.

16. Helen Fisher, "Broken Hearts: The Nature and Risk of Romantic Rejection," in *Romance and Sex in Adolescence and Emerging Adulthood: Risks and Opportunities*, ed. Ann C. Crouter and Alan Booth (Mahwah, NJ: Lawrence Erlbaum Associates, 2006), 19.

17. Daniel Wight, Alison Parkes, Vicki Strange, Elizabeth Allen, Chris Bonell, and Marion Henderson, "The Quality of Young People's Heterosexual Relationships: A Longitudinal Analysis of Characteristics Shaping Subjective Experience," *Perspectives on Sexual and Reproductive Health* 40 (2008).

18. Ibid.

19. Wyndol Furman and Laura Shaffer Hand, "The Slippery Nature of Romantic Relationships: Issues in Definition and Differentiation," in *Romance and Sex in Adolescence and Emerging Adulthood: Risks and Opportunities*, ed. Ann C. Crouter and Alan Booth (Mahwah, NJ: Lawrence Erlbaum Associates, 2006).

20. Laura Widman, Deborah P. Welsh, James K. McNulty, and Katherine C. Little, "Sexual Communication and Contraceptive Use in Adolescent Dating Couples," *Journal of Adolescent Health* 39, no. 6 (2006).

21. Monica Moore, "Courtship Signaling and Adolescents: 'Girls Just Wanna Have Fun'?" *Journal of Sex Research* 32, no. 4 (1995): 239.

22. L.M. Coleman and R. Ingham, "Exploring Young People's Difficulties in Talking about Contraception: How Can We Encourage More Discussion between Partners?" *Health Education Research* 14, no. 6 (1999).

23. Ibid., 474.

24. Susan Sprecher, Gardenia Harris, and Adena Meyers, "Perceptions of Sources of Sex Education and Targets of Sex Communication: Sociodemographic and Cohort Effects," *Journal of Sex Research* 45 (2008).

25. Heisler, "Family Communication about Sex," 306–7.

26. Schwartz et al., "What Elicits Romance," 53.

27. Ibid., 57.

28. Tricia M. Michels, Rhonda Y. Kropp, Stephen L. Eyre, and Bonnie L. Halpern-Felsher, "Initiating Sexual Experiences: How Do Young Adolescents Make Decisions Regarding Early Sexual Activity?" *Journal of Research on Adolescence* 15, no. 4 (2005): 596.

29. National Communication Association, "Interview with Dr. Claude Miller," in *Communication Currents*, ed. Joanne Keyton (Washington, DC: National Communication Association, 2009).

30. Centers for Disease Control and Prevention, "Adolescent Reproductive Health: Research," Centers for Disease Control and Prevention, http://www.cdc.gov/reproductivehealth/AdolescentReproHealth/Research.htm.

31. Laura Kann, "The Youth Risk Behavior Surveillance System: Measuring Health-Risk Behaviors," *American Journal of Health Behavior* 25, no. 3 (2001).

32. Michels et al., "Initiating Sexual Experiences."

33. Widman et al., "Sexual Communication and Contraceptive Use," 897.

34. Susan Donaldson James, "Study Reports Anal Sex on Rise among Teens: Lack of Sex Education, Virginity Pledges, Ignorance Contribute to Risky Behavior," http://abcnews.go.com/Health/story?id=6428003&page=1.

35. Wight et al., "Quality of Young Peoples Heterosexual Relationships."

CHAPTER 9
Sex and Health Communication

Bob had been experiencing back problems for a few years, but it has been much worse the last few weeks. He thinks he hurt his back lifting a chair but cannot be sure. It is affecting many aspects of his life: he cannot sit comfortably at work, he cannot sleep at night, and he is not interested in sex with his wife because he is afraid he will hurt his back even more. He made an appointment with his primary care provider and waited four days to get in to see her. He knows people who have had back surgery and the surgery led to even more back problems. Bob really hoped that it was not going to be a long-term problem and just wanted it to go away. He arrived to his doctor's appointment right on time but had to sit in the waiting room for 45 minutes. Bob figured this was OK since it was a last-minute appointment and four days is not terribly long to wait to talk to a doctor. His name was called and he was taken to a room where a nurse took his vitals and asked him why he came for the appointment. He waited another 15 minutes in this room for the doctor. When Dr. Jensen arrived, she asked him about his back, when it started to hurt, and to describe the pain. She did a five-minute exam of Bob's back and asked him to stretch and touch his toes. The entire time, Dr. Jensen was in charge of the questions, often cutting off Bob when she felt like she had heard enough to make an accurate diagnosis. She asked him a few questions about his back, wrote a prescription for a muscle relaxer, and referred him to a physical therapist. Dr. Jensen wished Bob the best and was in and out of the examination room in less than 15 minutes.

You probably have had both good and bad experiences at the doctor's office. All too often, people arrive early or on time to an appointment with a physician and are left in the waiting room before they are taken to an examination room to wait another 10 minutes to see the physician. By this time, most people are a bit irritated and feel like they should rush through their appointment because they have already spent enough time at the doctor's office, and they also realize that physicians are very busy. Unless the appointment is a yearly checkup, people visit the doctor for a specific concern. You probably state your concern or illness to the physician, just like Bob. The doctor arrives in the room, listens to you explain your symptoms, asks a few direct questions about the problem area, probably listens to your lungs or examines the part of your body that is causing the illness or hurts, writes a prescription and/or writes a referral, and then sends you off. Bob did not have a chance to talk to Dr. Jensen about any of the related issues of his back problem: the sleepless nights, problems at work, fears about long-term issues and surgery, and his lack of sex life. This is a communication problem. You probably feel like this is Dr. Jensen's fault, however, it is important to keep in mind that communication problems are rarely just one person's fault. It takes two to communicate, and this is especially important in the doctor's office.

INTRODUCTION

Research shows that economic factors, such as recession, do not affect people's sex drive. However, stress and insomnia do. A 2009 *Consumer Reports* poll of 1,000 people found that 81 percent of adults aged 18–75 reported avoiding or delaying sex with their partners in the past year.[1] The most common reasons that people reported for avoiding sex were tiredness (53%), illness (49%), and not being in the mood (40%). Fifty-six percent of men reported thinking about sex at least once daily versus only 19 percent of the women in the study. Obviously, many of these reasons are health related and could be addressed by medical professionals. Research also shows that most people would like to speak to their health care providers about their sexual health but do not know how. In this chapter, strategies to help people talk to physicians, nurses, and other health care providers about sexual issues are presented. Sex is one of the most important aspects of health and personal happiness, yet most people feel uncomfortable speaking with their health care providers about sex.

According to a report by medical doctor Charles Marwick, published in the *Journal of the American Medical Association*, over 85 percent of the adults polled indicated that they would like to talk to their physicians about sexual problems, but most do not. Approximately 71 percent said they thought their doctors would dismiss any concerns they might have, while 68 percent specifically stated they would not initiate sexuality issues because they thought it would embarrass their physicians. Regarding these issues, professor of clinical medicine at Columbia University's College of Physicians and Surgeons Marianee Lagato, an internationally known academic, physician, author, lecturer, and specialist in women's health, commented, "We need to establish an openness and level of comfort for Americans in speaking with their physicians and partners about sexual problems and health. Clearly sexual relations are of tremendous importance to the vast majority of the population, yet there remain inherent fears, misperceptions, and stigma about such issues."[2]

Women are not likely to talk to their doctors about sex; in a recent survey, more than half of the women polled never discussed sexually transmitted infections (STIs) with their doctors, and one in six kept sexual information from their providers.[3] In this same study, four out of five women underestimated or simply did not know the rates of STI infection in this country. It is estimated that as many as one in four Americans will get an STI at some point in their lifetimes. Just under half of women believed they would *know* if they had an STI, despite the fact that many STIs are asymptomatic. According to the Centers for Disease Control and Prevention, many of those who are infected don't know it.[4] And although most doctors acknowledged sexual health is extremely important and should be talked about with patients, few actually do it.[5]

Theoretically, it is the responsibility of health care professionals to inquire about sexual function; however, data suggest that very few physicians bring up sex and related issues with patients. A global survey assessed the importance of sexuality and intimacy in 26,000 men and women aged 40–80 in 29 countries. Surveys were completed by telephone or in a face-to-face interview. Only 14 percent of adults aged 40–80 years in the United States reported that a physician had asked about their sexual concerns within the past three years.[6] Another study involving a random-digit-dialed telephone opinion poll included 500 adults aged 25 years and older in the United States and surveyed reasons for patient reluctance to discuss sexual concerns. Seventy-one percent of people reported that they were reluctant to talk about sex with their doctors because they were afraid that that their concerns would be dismissed. Sixty-eight percent thought that their physicians would be uncomfortable, and 76 percent believed that there was a lack of treatment options (the doctor could not help them anyway).[7]

Sexuality experts Sheila MacNeil and Sandra Byers conducted an in-depth research project about communication with physicians about sex. They found that most participants did not seek out professional help even though they had a significant sexual concern or problem.[8] It is imperative to talk about sex with physicians because sex impacts numerous aspects of overall health and wellness. Yet patients do not expect their doctors to bring up sexual issues. Studies show that people are reluctant to bring up topics with their doctors such as bowel movements or sex organs because they think it is inappropriate. The importance of this extends beyond facilitating positive communicative encounters; many significant sexual health issues, such as STIs, need to be addressed in the clinical setting. Only 11 to 37 percent of primary care physicians routinely take a sexual history from new patients.[9] So it seems neither patients nor physicians are very good at addressing sexual health issues.

HEALTH CARE PROVIDER–PATIENT COMMUNICATION SKILLS

There has been a lot of research conducted and published regarding physicians' perspectives on communication and sex talk. Specifically, the bulk of this research focuses on identifying barriers to sexual talk in the doctor's office, suggesting curricula to train physicians, and providing talking points for physicians to improve their communication skills regarding sexual health issues. Some of the primary barriers that have been identified include the medicalization of sex in the clinical setting (focus on the biological dimensions of sex such as infertility, STIs, and erectile dysfunction) and the fact that most communication is health provider–driven and problem-based communication.[10] These barriers are discussed in this section in detail.

Historically, there has been a paternalistic relationship between doctors and patients. Because physicians were seen as more knowledgeable than patients and were believed ultimately to have the best interest of the patient in mind, patients were expected to cooperate and obey doctors' orders. Communication was one way: the doctor took the lead in the conversation and the patient was expected to follow. The paternalistic model has changed recently, and new forms of interaction between doctors and patients are being encouraged. Now many people realize the relationship should be more of a partnership; after all, 80 percent of a physician's diagnosis comes from taking a patient history.[11] Physicians need patients to be more involved in their own health care, to cooperate and adhere to medication regimes. To do this, a partnership must exist.

On a micro level, these shifts indicate that the medial community is aware of the need for better communication about sex between doctors and patients; however, given the constant stream of survey results that indicate doctors are still not addressing sex issues, it seems little of the information and/or impetus is trickling down into the actual office visit. The good news is that physicians are learning more about interpersonal communication, and a growing number of physicians are more comfortable talking about sex with their patients than ever before. Interpersonal communication skills have become policy in medical education, especially due to HIV/AIDS and other STIs. Realizing the importance for medical residents to possess and use effective communication skills, the American Council on Graduate Medical Education—the organization responsible for the accreditation of post-MD medical training programs within the United States—has explicitly identified interpersonal and communication skills as one of its six general competencies (the other five competencies include patient care, medical knowledge, practice-based learning and improvement, professionalism, and systems-based practice). The American Medical Association (AMA) has two policies addressing sex (H-170.966 "Human Sexuality Education" and H-75.994 "Contraception and Sexually Transmitted Diseases"), and these policies state that the AMA supports contraception and sex education.

Realistically, physician skills in talking about sex will vary. At the end of the day, physicians are normal people who get embarrassed or may feel uncomfortable talking about sex, especially if it is an area outside of their expertise. Some medical schools offer training on sexuality and sexual issues; however, some do not. Education and testing does not mean that new physicians will be comfortable talking about sex either. A physician who teaches in one of the largest medical schools in the country was telling me about a new physician he was training to specialize in infectious diseases, specifically treating people with HIV/AIDS and other STIs. This new physician could not ask his patients if they were sexually active.[12] One day, the teacher overheard the new doctor asking a patient if she had "social relations" instead of asking if she had sexual relations. He pulled the person aside and helped her understand the importance of taking a complete and accurate medical history and to appear to be comfortable doing so.

BARRIERS TO COMMUNICATION ABOUT SEX WITH PHYSICIANS

The sad reality is that doctors have a relatively short amount of time to make sometimes complex diagnoses when meeting with their patients. For most illnesses, identifying the cause of the problem is a process of elimination, so doctors need to collect specific information to narrow down their diagnoses. This is called *problem-solving communication*. Many illnesses have similar symptoms, and therefore many physicians are focused on gathering information about physical symptoms by asking specific questions about probable causes of the illness, while steering patients away from information that they consider to be unrelated to the condition so they can make an accurate diagnosis.[13] Physicians may not ask about important information for sensitive topics that may be relevant.

If a patient does not come in with a specific biological issue that affects his sexuality, such as contraception or STIs, physicians are probably not going to bring up any other topics regarding sex, particularly those that affect the psychosocial aspects of patients.[14] Physicians often underestimate patients' sexual concerns, especially because they find it difficult to address sexual health issues. Professional factors such as inadequate training and insufficient knowledge about sexual issues; time constraints; and even personal factors have been attributed to physician reluctance to discuss sex. Personal factors that influence a doctor's reluctance to talk about sex include conservative beliefs about sex, embarrassment, and the reluctance to intrude on a personal topic. Not surprisingly, a recent study found that doctors with more liberal beliefs about sex were more likely to bring up sex with patients, and this same study found that male physicians were much more liberal about sexual beliefs than female doctors.[15] In spite of how competent and helpful your doctor may be, talking about sex, especially specific risky sexual behaviors, can be tough. Your doctor may avoid talking about sex because she may worry about ruining the mutual trust the two of you have built.

Other changes in health care that have influenced doctor-patient communication are managed care (HMOs) and the Internet. In managed care, there are often strict time limits for which physicians are paid, and many physicians are forced to squeeze in more patients or even double-book appointments in case people do not show up. Because of time constraints, one can see how a doctor might become very focused on collecting specific information about a specific condition. Likewise, during a physical exam, doctors have a detailed checklist that they need to complete, and this often takes up the allotted appointment time. It does not mean that doctors are unwilling to talk about sexual issues, simply that it is not at the top of their agenda when they are meeting with patients. Therefore it is important for patients to help create a partnership and become more involved in their medical visits and voice any concerns they have. This is easier said than done. Reviewing lab results or discussing treatment options may leave little time for an adequate and helpful discussion about sex.

Even studies of women who have had genital track cancer, which significantly affects a woman's sexual organs and functions, found that doctors did not talk to the women about the ramifications of their illnesses on their sex lives.[16] Sexual problems resulting from the cancer included pain and lack of lubrication. "We found that these women valued sexuality and participated in sexual relationships and activities at a rate similar to women who had not been through cancer treatment, but they were not adequately prepared for the sexual issues that their cancer or its treatment introduced," study author Dr. Stacy Lindau said in a prepared statement about the study. Two out of three women whose reproductive and sexual organs were severely compromised by the treatment reported that their doctors never brought up sex. Lindau speculated that given the medical treatment on sexuality under these circumstances where it really counted, sexual health was even less likely to be discussed in other situations, particularly with older women.

The communication strategies that women used to talk to their doctors were investigated in a different study. A questionnaire was mailed to 1,584 women aged 18 years and older who received routine gynecological care at an army medical center. The survey instrument included 95 questions regarding sociodemographic characteristics, aspects of sexual history, sources of knowledge about sex, sexual concerns, and interest in and experience with discussing these sexual concerns with a physician. More than 90 percent of the participants reported that there were specific things that made it easier to discuss their sexual concerns with a doctor. If the physician seemed concerned, comfortable, kind, and understanding, then the women were much more likely to discuss sex. The women reported that physicians who maintained a professional demeanor made it much easier to talk to them. If the patient had seen the physician before and if the physician knew the patient were important factors. Approximately 60 percent of the participants did not feel that the physicians' gender influenced their discussions on sexual function. This study demonstrated that physicians' characteristics have an important impact on patients' comfort when discussing sexuality. Another study underscores the importance of physician-initiated questioning on sexuality.[17] This study found that it was really important for doctors to directly ask a patient if he had any sexual concerns. Only 3 percent of the patients spontaneously offered sexual complaints. With direct inquiry, 19 percent of the patients acknowledged a complaint.[18]

According to physicians, even when issues of sex are important and relevant, such as in the case of a cancer diagnosis, they often medicalize patients' sexuality and intimacy so that discussions remain at the level of patient fertility, contraception, erectile problems, or menopausal status.[19] Particularly in cancer situations, doctors said that it was a risky business to communicate about issues of patient intimacy and sexuality after cancer. In addition, health professionals often make assumptions about patients' sexuality based on the patient's age, diagnosis, culture, partnership, and disease status and rarely check to see if these assumptions are true.

COMMUNICATION ABOUT SEX BETWEEN DOCTORS AND ADOLESCENTS

It has been observed that physician discussions with adolescents about sexual risks reduce adolescent risk-taking behaviors. Physicians are an excellent source of accurate medical information about sex for teens for many reasons. First, most adolescents see a physician at least once a year, and most young adolescents indicate a desire for information on sexuality from their physicians. Finding someone to whom teens want to talk about sex and who has accurate information is difficult enough, so the fact that teens actually want to talk to doctors is a positive indicator.

However, when it comes to sex talk, numerous issues make it more difficult and uncomfortable for both teens and doctors to talk. Certain topics, such as sexual problems and STIs, are particularly difficult to address. There are many barriers that prevent teens from talking with their doctors about sex. Confidentiality, particularly from parents, is an important issue to most adolescents and a major reason why some may not seek care from their physicians for a sexual problem. For example, a study involving 221 young adolescents aged 12–15 years that assessed their comfort discussing sexual problems with their physicians revealed some significant barriers.[20] Approximately 89 percent of teens said that they valued their physicians' opinions about sex, and 99 percent said it was easy to talk to the physician during their visit. Almost half said they would be uncomfortable talking to the physician if they had a STI or some other sexual problem (43%). Adolescents' sense of comfort was greater in certain situations. When physicians discussed sexual issues in the general health examination, when adolescents perceived their personal risk of sexually transmitted disease to be high, if adolescents had high self-esteem, and when physicians were adolescents' usual physicians greatly increased the comfort and likelihood that teens would talk to their doctors. The burden for initiating sexual discussions really falls upon the doctor because about 50 percent of adolescents report that they would not seek care related to sexual concerns from their physicians. Parents can specifically ask their teens' doctors to bring up the topic of sex to make sure that doctors do it.

Almost all adolescents reported that it was easy talking with the physician during their general health visit, that they were comfortable talking to the physician, and that they believed that the physician cared about them as people. A little over half of female adolescents said they would be comfortable talking to the physician if they had an STI or some other sexual problem. The majority of girls (63%) indicated that they would be much more comfortable talking to a woman physician. Only 39 percent of girls said they would be comfortable talking to a male physician. Boys did not really differ in levels of comfort when it came to physician gender. Among girls, comfort was greater the more thoroughly the physician spoke about sexual issues. This was also true for the younger teens: 12- to 13-year-old adolescents felt much more comfortable when doctors were thorough and direct in their discussions about sex. Higher perceived susceptibility to STI infection was associated with greater sense of comfort among male adolescents only. Self-esteem also played an important role: among female adolescents and 12- to 13-year-olds, the greater the self-esteem, the greater their sense of comfort. One thing is clear from this study: with age comes comfort. The older boys became, the more comfortable they felt when talking to doctors about sexual problems. Boys aged 14 and 15 years were more likely to say they would be comfortable talking to the physician about a sexual problem than those who were aged 12–13 years.

What do adolescents talk about with their doctors? The most commonly talked about topics were pubertal changes (69%), STIs (68%), sex (63%), HIV infection and AIDS (57%), and condoms (51%).

Unfortunately, fewer than half of the adolescents in this study said that the physicians discussed pregnancy protection (48%), delaying sexual intercourse (36%), limiting one's number of partners (19%), using a condom correctly (17%), nonpenetrative sexual activities (7%), and masturbation (6%). When adolescents reported that the physician talked to them about HIV infection and AIDS, condoms, delaying sexual intercourse, limiting one's number of partners, and using a condom correctly during the general health visit, they were more likely to feel comfortable talking to the physician if they had a sexual problem in the future. Over three-fourths of adolescents trusted that the physician would maintain confidentiality about their sexual behavior.[21]

Most adolescents in this study said they highly valued physicians' opinions about sex. Almost all adolescents were comfortable talking to the physician during their general health visit, and most adolescents thought that the physician cared about them as people. Nevertheless, almost half of the adolescents indicated that they would not be comfortable talking to the physician if they had an STI or some other sexual problem. Such discomfort may be a reason why previous studies show that adolescents are reluctant to seek care for sexual problems from their primary care physicians.

While most adolescents in this study reported that the physician talked to them about puberty and STIs, few adolescents reported that their physicians talked to them about specific ways of reducing sexual risks. The more physicians discussed sexual risks and protection measures (including abstinence) with these adolescents, the greater their sense of comfort talking to the physicians about sexual problems. Because fewer than half of the adolescents received specific sexual risk prevention messages from the physician, the researchers suggested that physicians more often and more thoroughly discuss these topics with all young adolescents. Physicians may make their adolescent patients more comfortable seeking care for sexual problems if they clearly discuss and clarify their policies on confidentiality, particularly on what will and will not be shared with parents. Again, parents can ask their children's physicians to specifically address sexual risk prevention strategies to ensure the topic is covered during a visit.

Another barrier to physician and other health care provider communication, particularly among adolescents, is one of vocabulary. Oftentimes, doctors use medical terms for sex terminology that adolescents do not understand; likewise, teens have their own language for sex acts unfamiliar to physicians. For example, a study with 41 males and 157 females aged 9–19 years showed that there were several possible misunderstandings by adolescents of common medical terms (e.g., penile discharge) and some words were not known, or synonyms could not be provided, by some adolescents for terms such as vulva/labia.[22] Also, teens used some slang terms to refer to more than one sexual term, perhaps owing to lack of knowledge. It is obvious that teens use different terminology with their friends than they do with their physicians; however, this could lead to many misunderstandings between physicians and teens.

In another study in California that examined teen communication with doctors about sex, about 39 percent of the high school students in the study reported discussions with physicians about how to avoid getting AIDS from sex, 37 percent discussed condom use for vaginal intercourse, 13 percent talked about how to use condoms, 15 percent talked about the adolescent's sex life, 13 percent addressed strategies to say no to unwanted sex, and 8 percent spoke about sexual orientation.[23] Around 8 percent of the teens said they had been given a condom by a doctor. This study found that 80–90 percent of the teens in the study said they would find it at least a little helpful to talk with a physician about sexual issues. Most would trust a physician to keep secret and not tell their parents if they asked questions about sex (75%), indicated that they were having sex (65%), or confided that they were using contraception (68%). However, a smaller number would trust physicians to keep secret a STI (44%) or pregnancy (44%). For adolescents who knew that physicians in California do not have to tell parents about STIs or pregnancy, levels of trust rose to a mere 54 percent. It is concerning that most doctors do not bring up sex issues with adolescents even though polls show that doctors feel adolescents are among the highest risk groups for STIs.

MATURE PATIENTS

Physicians often bring societal age and gender biases to their perceptions regarding which patients are sexually active (and therefore possibly at risk for the heterosexual transmission of HIV and other STIs) that influence their communication about sexual health issues with older patients. Primary care physicians may mistakenly conclude that sexual issues are unimportant to divorced or widowed mature patients, especially women. A 2007 study in the *New England Journal of Medicine* reported that the prevalence of sexual activity declined with age and that women were significantly less likely than men at all ages to report sexual activity. Among older respondents who were sexually active, about half of both men and women reported at least one bothersome sexual problem. The most prevalent sexual problems among women were low desire (43%), difficulty with vaginal lubrication (39%), and inability to climax (34%). Around 37 percent of men said they had erectile difficulties, which were the most prevalent sexual problems for men. Yet only 14 percent of all men reported using medication or supplements to improve sexual function. Men and women who rated their health as being poor were less likely to be sexually active and, among respondents who were sexually active, were more likely to report sexual problems. A total of 38 percent of men and 22 percent of women reported having discussed sex with a physician since the age of 50. The interesting thing about this study is that researchers found that even though almost half of men and women aged 57–85 had at least one sexual problem, only 38 percent of men and 22 percent of women over 50 years of age discussed sex with their doctors.[24]

Although research suggests that many single mature people are sexually active, physicians are often reluctant to discuss sexual matters with them. In a study of recently single women aged 45–68, 64 percent of them believed that they were at risk for HIV and STIs. Most physicians reported that they believe younger patients to be most at risk for STIs and that risk declined with patients' advancing age and with female status. Doctors seem to be much more likely to discuss sexual matters with mature men. Sexual health issues are relevant to mature women's continued health and well-being and yet are often ignored by doctors.

As patients get older, physicians are less likely to speak with them about sexual issues. Old age does not diminish sex drive, and it has been shown that when older people are not involved in a sexually intimate relationship, it is due to lack of a partner rather than a lack of desire for sex.[25] The level of sexual activity in nursing homes is surprising to most people. Given the fact that a nursing home is pretty much a co-ed home with close quarters and is occupied by people with lots of free time, it seems natural for people to form intimate relationships. Most of the literature and popular press about sexual relationships in nursing homes treats sex among the elderly as inappropriate; however, it is occurring at increasing rates.[26] Children who have a parent in a nursing home have a particularly difficult time accepting the fact that their parents might be sexually active and refuse to sign consent forms for contraceptives. Condom use is encouraged in nursing homes given the risk of STIs in these situations.

DO YOU NEED A MEDICAL SPECIALIST?

There are situations in which referral to a sex therapist can be helpful in treating sexual dysfunction. In many cases, collaboration between physician and sex therapist may be necessary for successful treatment. Sexual dysfunctions that have been long standing or lifelong are often associated with anger, performance anxiety, and sex avoidance behavior. When people have more than one dysfunction, it may be difficult for the physician to identify the initial cause of sexual problems, and a specialist might be needed. The specialist can be medical, such as a urologist, or psychological. Psychological problems, such as depression, anxiety, interpersonal problems, current or past sexual abuse, and substance abuse, have a negative impact on sexual function and complicate treatment strategies.

Finally, you may need to see a specialist if you have a lack of response to regularly prescribed medicines to treat the problem. Sex therapists typically have an advanced degree in social work, medicine, or psychology and have undergone specialized training in human sexuality. Certification is not necessary but can be obtained by the American Association of Sex Educators, Counselors, and Therapists or the American Board of Sexology. Sex therapists with certification must participate in continuing education and adhere to a code of ethics. There are Web sites of these organizations that can serve as resources for identifying sex therapists. Also, asking your primary care physician for a referral is usually a way to get a qualified, board-certified specialist.

HOW TO TALK TO YOUR DOCTOR ABOUT SEX

From what all the research says, it looks like it is really up to the patient to get the conversation started with a doctor. There are a few things that people can do to help the process along. Try to give the doctor the benefit of the doubt and start the conversation yourself. In fact, numerous studies involving doctor-patient communication about sex show that most doctors are not going to bring up the topic of sexual satisfaction with patients, so it is often up to the patient to initiate the conversation. If time is a serious issue, you may need to make a follow-up appointment dedicated to talking about your sexual concerns and get a complete medical workup. Also, talk to your doctor about whether you should go directly to a specialist. You should do this if you get the feeling your doctor is uncomfortable talking about sex with you or you are uncomfortable with her. Many people prefer to talk to same-sex physicians. You can request a same-sex specialist with whom to talk about your issues.

TIPS TO START THE CONVERSATION

Researchers at the University of San Francisco Center for Health Improvement and Prevention Studies offer tips to help patients talk to their doctors about sex.[27] In the end, it is up to you, the consumer:

- Make sure you are dressed and not on the examination table when you start a discussion.[28] You should really do this with any discussion.

- Plan before you go. Doctors tend to interrupt patients early on when they are trying to talk about their concerns, so think about what you'd like to ask, and see if you can put it into a question that is one or two sentences. You can fill in the details afterward.

- Ask about confidentiality. Doctors are required to keep communication with patients confidential, but it doesn't mean they always will. It's a good idea to ask your doctor what the rules of confidentiality are and to let him know that you want the conversation to be private, even if your doctor also sees your spouse or partner as a patient.

- Be prepared for her discomfort. We tend to project a lot of expectations on our doctors. But like anyone else, your doctor may be uncomfortable talking about sex with you. This doesn't mean that you can't do it, and it doesn't mean that your doctor can't be helpful to you. Being prepared for a little bit of awkwardness will guard against you backing out at the last minute.

- If you are too embarrassed to start the conversation, hand your doctor a note with your questions and say, "Here are some questions I would like to have answered or addressed today."

- Before your doctor breaks into his routine, help set the agenda for your appointment. You might start the conversation by saying, "I have some concerns about my sex life. Could we take some time today to discuss them?" Your initiative can guide your doctor to prioritize your sexual concerns.

- If your doctor dances around the topic of sex, you can reframe the discussion and steer the conversation to one that meets your needs. You can say, "How can I stay healthy and have sex?"

- Remember to encourage your doctor in talking about sex. You might say, "I am glad we are talking about sex. I appreciate your suggestions."

- Share your life's realities with your doctor. This may mean opening up to him about the behavior and attitudes of people around you that make it tough to stay safe. Naming your obstacles will help your doctor better support you in staying healthy.

- If you hear your doctor repeat the same advice time after time, consider it proof of her caring about you. Such words of concern can make a big difference.

- Try to do your own research online or in the library to learn more about what sexual practices are considered safe and unsafe and what you can do to protect yourself and others. After the research, you may have further questions to discuss with your doctor. Taking charge of information and news sources can ensure that you obtain the best care possible.

- Keep the door open for further discussions. Ask your doctor if he would be willing to take more time to discuss sex with you at your next appointment or whether he could refer you to another member of the health care team who can help.

- Consider talking to a nurse. Patients often overlook these excellent sources of medical knowledge about sex. Many nurses share the perceptions that patients do not expect nurses to address their sexuality concerns and therefore are reluctant to bring issues up. However, if you bring the topic up, you might be surprised at how informed and friendly nurses can be.[29]

- Consider talking to friends. Only pick people you think will respect your privacy and can handle a serious conversation about sex. Doing this can give you valuable information about other people's experiences and may also give you practice in talking about your concerns.

NOTES

1. Consumer Reports Health Poll, "80% of Sexually Active Americans Put Off Sex Because They're Too Sick or Tired," *Consumer Reports*, http:// pressroom.consumerreports.org/pressroom/2009/02/consumer-reports-

health-poll-80-of-sexually-active-americans-put-off-sex-because-theyre-too-sick-or-.html.

2. Charles Marwick, "Survey Says Patients Expect Little Physician Help on Sex," *Journal of the American Medical Association* 281 (1999): 2173.

3. Tina Hoff, Andrea Miller, Jennifer Barefoot, and Liberty Greene, "National Survey of Women about Their Sexual Health: Take Charge of Your Sexual Health," Kaiser Family Foundation, http://www.kff.org/women shealth/20030618a-index.cfm.

4. Centers for Disease Control and Prevention, "Adolescent Reproductive Health: Research," Centers for Disease Control and Prevention, http://www.cdc.gov/reproductivehealth/AdolescentReproHealth/Research.htm.

5. N.H.J. Haboubi and N. Lincoln, "Views of Health Professionals on Discussing Sexual Issues with Patients," *Disability and Rehabilitation* 25, no. 6 (2003).

6. Edward Laumann, Anthony Paik, Dale B. Glasser, Jeong-Han Kang, Tianfu Wang, Bernard Levinson, Edson Moreira, Alfredo Nicolosi, and Clive Gingel, "The Pfizer Global Study of Sexual Attitudes and Behaviors," Pfizer, http://www.pfizerglobalstudy.com/study/study-results.asp.

7. Marwick, "Survey Says Patients Expect Little Physician Help on Sex."

8. Sheila MacNeil and E. Sandra Byers, "The Relationships between Sexual Problems, Communication, and Sexual Satisfaction," *Canadian Journal of Human Sexuality* 6, no. 4 (1997). There were 87 men and women in the study.

9. American Medical Association Council on Scientific Affairs, "Health Care Needs of Gay Men and Lesbians in the United States," *Journal of the American Medical Association* 275, no. 17 (1996).

10. Leonore Tiefer, "Sexual Behaviour and Its Medicalisation. Many (Especially Economic) Forces Promote Medicalisation," *British Medical Journal* 325, no. 7354 (2002).

11. See Robert E. Rakel, *Textbook of Family Practice*, 6th ed. (Maryland Heights, MO: MD Consult, 2002), 247.

12. Hans Schlecht, personal communication, June 12, 2009.

13. Kevin Wright, Lisa Sparks, and Dan O'Hair, *Health Communication in the 21st Century* (Malden, MA: Blackwell, 2008).

14. Stamatis Papaharitou, Evangelia Nakopoulou, Martha Moraitou, Zoi Tsimtsiou, Eleni Konstantinidou, and Dimitrios Hatzichristou, "Exploring Sexual Attitudes of Students in Health Professions," *Journal of Sexual Medicine* 5, no. 6 (2008).

15. Ibid.

16. Stacy Lindau, Natalia Gavrilova, and David Anderson, "Sexual Morbidity in Very Long Term Survivors of Vaginal and Cervical Cancer: A Comparison to National Norms," *Gynecologic Oncology* 106, no. 2 (2007).

17. G. A. Bachmann, S. R. Leiblum, and J. Grill, "Brief Sexual Inquiry in Gynecologic Practice," *Obstetrics and Gynecology* 73, no. 3, Pt. 1 (1989).

18. Ibid.

19. A.J. Hordern and A.F. Street, "Let's Talk about Sex: Risky Business for Cancer and Palliative Care Clinicians," *Contemporary Nurse* 27, no. 1 (2007).

20. B.O. Boekeloo, L.A. Schamus, T.L. Cheng, and S.J. Simmens, "Young Adolescents' Comfort with Discussion about Sexual Problems with Their Physician," *Archives of Pediatrics and Adolescent Medicine* 150, no. 11 (1996).

21. Seventy-seven percent among 12- and 13-year-olds and 88% among 14- and 15-year-olds.

22. M.S. Barratt and W.L. Risser, "Sexual Terminology: A Barrier to Communication between Adolescents and Health Care Providers," *Ambulatory Child Health* 4, no. 1 (1998).

23. M.A. Schuster, R.M. Bell, L.P. Petersen, and D.E. Kanouse, "Communication between Adolescents and Physicians about Sexual Behavior and Risk Prevention," *Archives of Pediatrics and Adolescent Medicine* 150, no. 9 (1996).

24. Stacy Tessler Lindau, L. Philip Schumm, Edward O. Laumann, Wendy Levinson, Colm A. O'Muircheartaigh, and Linda J. Waite, "A Study of Sexuality and Health among Older Adults in the United States," *New England Journal of Medicine* 357, no. 8 (2007).

25. D. Kuhn, "Intimacy, Sexuality, and Residents with Dementia," *Alzheimer's Care Quarterly* 3, no. 2 (2002).

26. Ibid., 166.

27. Barbara Gerbert, Dale Danley, Dung Huynh, Daniel Ciccarone, Paul Gilbert, David Bangsberg, Kathleen Clanon, Anas Hana, and Michael Allerton, *Bet You and Your Doctor Don't Talk about Sex: A Conversation Starter for HIV-Positive Men and Women* (San Francisco: University of California Center for Health Improvement and Prevention Studies).

28. J. Tomlinson, "ABC of Sexual Health: Taking a Sexual History," *British Medical Journal* 317, no. 7172 (1998).

29. M.A. Magnan and K. Reynolds, "Barriers to Addressing Patient Sexuality Concerns across Five Areas of Specialization," *Clinical Nurse Specialist* 20, no. 6 (2006).

CHAPTER 10

The Dark Side of Sexual Relationships: Communication Is Not a Cure-All

There is a potential dark side to communication about sex: deception, relational transgression, risk, disclosure of sexually transmitted infection (STI) status, taboo topics, sexual addiction, and pornography, to name a few. What if you disclose a fantasy and your partner rejects it? How do we know when and what to disclose? How do we talk to our partners about personal issues such as cheating? What happens when a partner starts to hate the characteristics and communication choices that supposedly attracted her to a person in the first place?

There is statistical evidence about the factors that make some marriages prone to divorce: age at the time of marriage (the younger people are when they get married, the more likely they are to divorce), education (people with lower levels of education are more likely to divorce), ethnicity (blacks have the highest rate of divorce, followed by whites and Hispanics; Asians have the lowest rates), and remarriage (people who have been divorced before are more likely to divorce again; approximately 50% of people in first marriages divorce, compared to 60% in second marriages).[1] This chapter does not focus on many of these causes; rather a review of communication and relational issues that are associated with breakups is provided.

Sociologist Diane Felmlee's research findings led her to conclude that often, what first attracted people to someone is likely to be the thing that repels them at the end of the relationship. "Like a moth to a flame, individuals are drawn to the very aspects of another individual that they eventually dislike."[2] The boyfriend that a woman fell in love with because he was so much fun now drives her nuts because he is irresponsible and silly. The girlfriend that was so successful and organized and had it all together is now controlling and inflexible. Felmlee examines how attraction turns to disillusionment in her research. She believes that vices and virtues are one and the same and that a quality or trait that someone initially finds attractive can turn into annoying in the flash of an eye—based on changes in personal perception, relational dynamics and tensions, and circumstances. To some extent, disillusionment is a natural occurrence due to the naturally occurring ebbs and flows of the needs of individuals in a couple. Recall that there are ongoing tensions in relationships; people want connection and autonomy and move through phases where they want more of one than the other. Remember that relationships are fluid and ever changing, and so are circumstances in life. You make have liked the fact that you are married to a hard worker, a person devoted to providing a better life for the family and children; however, this person might not be much fun when the kids are out of the house and couples are facing 20 plus years of retirement together.

Felmlee theorized that there are several specific reasons why disillusionment occurs. She believes that at the beginning of relationships, people tend to focus on the positive traits of a person and ignore or downplay the negative characteristics and annoying communication habits of people. Over time, the likelihood of ignoring annoying traits diminishes and people see something that was always there to begin with. She also believes that the old saying "familiarity breeds contempt" is an apt explanation of what happens between couples: what was once attractive is no longer. Simply put, it gets old. Also, reinforcement can amplify a behavior and excess can make it annoying. If you constantly compliment your partner on his sense of humor and tell him that is what drew you to him in the first place, then he may start to tell jokes excessively in an effort to please you, but the excess drives you nuts, until you reach the point that you cannot hear one more joke. It is easy to relate to all of these explanations and the theory that eventually, inevitably, some of the things that attracted us to a person in the first place are the very things we cannot stand at the end of a relationship.

Couples that have a significant imbalance of power tend to divorce more than those who have more equality in their relationships. For almost all couples, there is an imbalance of equality in a relationship. One person has more relational power than the other, and oftentimes the person with more power fluctuates over the course of a relationship. However, research showed that for marriages when power in the relationship is more equal, marital satisfaction of both parties is higher. Communication scholars Laura Guerrero, Angela La Valley, and Lisa

Farinelli completed a study that examined how expressions of anger, guilt, and sadness are related to inequity and marital satisfaction.[3] They interviewed 92 couples and found that some overbenefited from the marriage; this means they got more from the marriage than they were contributing. The majority of people who overbenefited from the marriage felt guilty. The underbenefited, those who were contributing more to the marriage than they were getting back, were significantly more angry and depressed than their spouses. Underbenefited wives also reported high levels of sadness. People who perceived equity in their relationships reported using more constructive, prosocial emotional communication: communicating love and respect for partners, both verbally and nonverbally. Not surprisingly, underbenefited people reported using more destructive, antisocial emotional communication. Interestingly, overbenefited people reported using positive, prosocial, and antisocial emotional expressions. Both husbands and wives reported higher levels of marital satisfaction when they perceived themselves to be treated equitably or to be overbenefited as compared to underbenefited. In the end, the researchers found that angry feelings and aggressive expressions of anger were the result of perceived unequal power in relationships.

In 1994, communication scholars William Cupach and Brian Spitzberg published a book called *The Dark Side of Interpersonal Communication*; in 1998, they published a follow-up to that volume called *The Dark Side of Close Relationships*. In these books, they explain that most research and writings that address relationships in general and, more specially, communication paint an unrealistically happy picture of the world. They write, "[The] original impetus [for our book] was the belief that the social sciences were overly pollyanna-like in perspective," evidenced clearly in "the contents of most undergraduate textbooks, littered with commendations to be attractive, open, honest, self-confident, assertive, visionary, good-humored, supportive, cooperative, empathic, clear, polite, competent, and to develop and maintain normal friendships, heterosexual romances, and resilient nuclear families."[4] They provide compelling evidence that relationships are not that simple. Communication is not that simple either. They provide research that shows that "attractiveness can be a curse, openness can be costly, honesty is often more destructive than deceit, self-esteem can be self-absorbing and a source of aggression, assertiveness tends to be unlikable, visionary leadership can be misguided, humor can be violent and oppressive, supportiveness can aggravate rather than heal, cooperation and empathy are susceptible to exploitation," and so on.[5] For every aspect of communication presented in this text and others, there are ways in which it can backfire and has been shown to do so in research. Communication can and does go wrong, even when it is done right. However, Cupach and Spitzberg claim that acknowledging and, more important, understanding the dark side of interpersonal communication can help people be more cautious overall and less likely to put up with unchecked abuse through interpersonal communication. After all, they argue, a holistic approach to relationships requires an understanding of the entire relational system, including the darker aspects.[6]

Spitzberg and Cupach illuminate the metaphor of the dark side by claiming that there are many types of darknesses to explore. They identify and explain seven darknesses that are particularly applicable to interpersonal communication, and I relate each of these to communication about sex. First, there is the darkness concerned with the "dysfunctional, distorted, distressing, and destructive aspects of human action."[7] This darkness is so harmful that it can eventually lessen one's ability to function. In terms of communication about sex, it is easy to see how this occurs and is destructive to so many sexual relationships, especially if the gender roles and influence of the media are examined. Chapter 2 explored the ways in which media distort our reality of sexual relationships and not only limit modeling of meaningful sex talk, but actively discourage it. Showing such distorted images and depictions of sexual relationships can greatly alter one's realistic expectations of what to expect in a relationship and how to talk about sex. Furthermore, in chapter 3, it was clear that culturally determined gender roles not only silenced important talk about sex but made it very difficult for women to flip a switch at marriage and suddenly become fully sexual beings after years of oppressing desires and acting as sexual gatekeepers against men.

Second, there is the darkness concerned with the "deviance, betrayal, transgression, and violation."[8] This is communication that is awkward, rude, disruptive, and annoying. Spitzberg and Cupach remind readers that we have been acculturated to behave and communicate in certain ways, mostly to ensure societal continuity and comfort. Violations of these norms can be extremely harmful. When we learn that people are supposed to talk a certain way in close relationships or act a certain way in sexual relationships, it is extremely harmful when norms are broken. Take self-disclosure about sex, for example. Most of how we disclose sexual information is based on societal norms, and people have expectations about how, when, where, why, and to whom it is appropriate to disclose. It is inappropriate to disclose personal information too soon in a relationship; likewise, disclosure is expected as the relationship progresses. If a person breaks the communicative norms involving sexual self-disclosure, it can lead to the end of a relationship or may prevent some people from ever even entering into a close personal relationship.

"Third, the dark side is concerned with the exploitation of the innocent. . . . Harming those who have little power to protect themselves from harm is another source of darkness." As noted in chapter 7, there are different power levels in a relationship. Those that take advantage of another person in a sexual relationship definitely fall into this dark side of communication. Fourth, the dark side is concerned with the "unfulfilled, unpotentiated, underestimated, and unappreciated human endeavors."[9] This refers to lost loves and loves never found, regrets, and ruminations about those regrets.

Fifth, the dark side is "concerned with the unattractive, unwanted, distasteful, and repulsive." Sixth is the dark side dealing with objectification. "The treatment of people's basic humanity as if inhuman, diminishing a person's personhood, and categorically reducing an individual to the status of thing are all ways of deanimating humans."[10] Communicating about sex for those who society has deemed unattractive is particularly difficult as it is difficult for them to find a partner in the first place. Recall the study in chapter 6 about the research experiment involving two men who used the exact same communication strategies on single women. One was considered attractive and the other was unattractive. The communication strategies that the good-looking man employed with women were deemed "cute and sexy" by women, but these same lines were deemed "annoying and repulsive" by women when the unattractive man tried them out. It is especially difficult for people to navigate interpersonal relationships when they have been identified as unwanted by the majority of people in a society.

Seventh, and finally, is the darkness concerned with the "paradoxical, dialectical, dualistic, and mystifying aspects of life."[11] Consider the work by Felmlee. An example of this is in the paradox between people's relationship statuses and likelihood to have safe sex. It is paradoxical that being in a relationship has been shown to both decrease and increase a person's risk for STIs. Research has shown that people in a relationship are more trusting of a person and therefore more comfortable skipping condom use because they trust their partner. At the same time, because of the increased comfort level, people in a relationship have been shown to talk about and have safe sex more because they trust their partner. There are strong connections between sexual intimacy in relationships and relational commitment; by extension, the issue of fidelity as part of relational commitment is implicated. Commitment leads to comfort and trust, and therefore partners are more likely to feel at ease discussing sexual issues and engaging in safer sex practices. On the other hand, commitment leads to trust, and therefore partners feel like they do not have to practice safer sex because of the very fact that they trust their partners. Furthermore, numerous studies highlight that relational commitment, and specifically relational commitment to an ideal of monogamy, actually leads to unsafe sex practices and HIV risk denial.

Spitzberg and Cupach concluded that some issues are more serious than others; however, it is important not to underestimate the devastating effects of "the lifetimes of quiet struggle, dissatisfaction, and sense of frustration, anger, and despair that result from merely suboptimal forms of human endeavor in our significant (and even mundane) relationships with others."[12] It is essential to remember that interpersonal communication can both cause quiet desperation and cure it.

MORE ON THE DARK SIDE: COMMUNICATIVE RESPONSES TO JEALOUSY

Most scholars acknowledge that there are positive and negative aspects to jealousy. On the positive side, jealousy can "show love and appreciation, add romance to a dull relationship, or help one realize the extent and care of commitment he or she feels for another."[13] The negative consequences are far reaching and serious in that jealousy can be problematic for interpersonal relationships; jealous feelings are indicative of relational dissatisfaction, and when jealousy is severe, it can lead to abusive and violent behavior. How people handle and respond to jealousy largely determines whether the relational outcome will be negative or positive.

There are various communicative responses to jealousy, and these fall into two categories: interactive responses and general behavior responses. The first category is called the *interactive response*. This response to jealousy "entails communication, typically face to face, that is directed toward the partner, although in some instances it may involve avoiding interaction with the partner."[14] Displays of nonverbal expression of jealousy-induced emotions such as depression, anger, or frustration are commonly directed to the partner. These are often expressed involuntarily. Specifically, these responses range from what the researchers call *integrative communication*, which is prosocial communication involving rational communication with a partner, to *distributive communication*, which is largely antisocial and involves accusing a partner and yelling rather than engaging in a calm conversation. Another possible response is active distancing, where a person avoids interaction with a partner and does not display affection to the partner. Avoidance and/or denial are when the jealous person becomes quiet and denies feelings of jealousy. Unfortunately, some responses result in violent communication, where the jealous partner physically harms the other or threatens to do harm. Jealousy may cause a person to communicate in any of these ways.

The second category of responses are called *general behavior responses*, which are communication based but are unlikely to occur face-to-face. These responses involve spying. The jealous person may try to restrict access and interaction between the rival and his partner. Another possible response in this category that does not involve direct communication is simply an effort made by the jealous person to improve the relationship and make staying in the relationship more attractive to her partner. Essentially, the person attempts to make herself look like the best partner for the other person. A separate response that is along this line is to try to make the rival look bad by denigrating the rival. The partner may seek revenge by trying to make the other person jealous or feel guilty. Another possible response is for the person to contact the rival person to gain information about the person and the rival relationship or to discourage the rival from being interested in his partner. The jealous person may indicate that the person is taken and not on the market to the rival. Violence is also a potential occurrence, but in the category of general behavior responses, it is limited to violence against objects such as throwing something or slamming a door. As a last resort, a person may threaten to end the relationship or to have an affair with another person if her jealous feelings are not addressed.

It has been shown that jealous people tend to use a variety of communicative responses and often end up using a combination of destructive and constructive communication.[15] It is tough to know when to confront someone who is jealous. It is also tough to be the jealous person and know when to confront a partner because most people do not want to seem jealous or insecure. However, avoiding confrontation may be more harmful to the relationship than keeping quiet because it may leave the person with feelings of uncertainly about the relationship and cause him to ruminate over the state of the relationship unnecessarily, leading to relational dissatisfaction.[16] *Rumination* is when someone thinks too much and worries about the security of the relationship. Rumination is distressing and tends to perpetuate itself. Jealousy can have a positive effect on the relationship if it encourages someone to improve the relationship through positive methods such as increased affectionate communication or participation in chores. However, often, people are uncertain as to whether their efforts are working to improve the relationship because their partners do not give them adequate feedback, so this can be a frustrating response, as well. Researchers also found that some people go out of their way not to seek information about a possible rival because they are so scared of losing the relationship.

The researchers conclude that the tactics a person uses to confront a partner about a rival largely depend on how the person thinks his partner is going to respond: either confirming his suspicions or denying them. They found that if a jealous person thinks his partner will deny the charges, then he will use integrative communication. If the person expects his partner to confirm the charges, then he will use a strategy that either attacks or creates distance.[17]

TALKING ABOUT PORNOGRAPHY
WITH YOUR PARTNER

Pornography is a hot topic; many books and articles have been written that offer perceptive analyses of how pornography affects interpersonal relationships and how men and women are viewed in our culture. The word *pornography* is Greek in origin, deriving from *porno* (prostitute) and *graphein* (to write). Many researchers differentiate pornography from erotica. *Erotica* is sexually graphic material that portrays sex as an equal activity between partners involving mutually sensual pleasure rather than images of power and subordination.[18] The term *pornography* is invoked when images degrade or demean people. Of course, this is a matter of opinion. Two people can watch the same movie, where one finds it degrading to women and the other does not; at the end of the day, it is a matter of opinion.

Because defining *pornography* is such an individually based effort, I suggest that you speak to your partner about it as you would speak about any taboo topic. Approach your partner calmly, perhaps with a self-disclosure, and seek compromises that result in both of you being happy. Since erotica has been shown to benefit some people's sex lives,[19] perhaps a discussion about how each individual thinks about pornography and erotica is a good starting point. An end point would be making efforts to move a partner to material that both people consider erotica.

CHEATING

In the National Health and Social Life Survey, Dr. Laumann and colleagues reported that 24.5 percent of men and 15 percent of women in the United States have experienced extramarital sex.[20] Sociologist Chien Liu set out to find out why the frequency of sex decreases as the length of marriage increases and if this really does motivate people to cheat. One might think, "Oh, the obvious answer to a decline in sexual frequency is because people are aging and getting older," but research has shown that duration and age have the same negative impacts on sexual frequency. Think about it this way: two couples that have both been married for 15 years will have roughly the same decrease in sex—even though one couple was married at 20 years of age (they now are 35 years old) and the other couple was married at 40 years of age (they now are 55 years old). Another commonly cited reason for a decease in sexual frequency, especially in popular culture, is the belief that sex becomes less exciting when the novelty wears off and people get bored with the same sex, often referred to as the honeymoon effect. However, rational choice theory directly opposes the hypothesis of the honeymoon effect and states that people in long-term relationships are more committed to partner pleasing, and research supports the claim that sex is better in marriages. There is no empirical proof that people become bored with the same sexual routine. However, it makes sense that there are a limited number of new and novel techniques and ideas that one can incorporate into a sexual relationship, so there are fewer and fewer acceptable and pleasing options to spice up sex over time. From an economic standpoint, when people have children, their resource allocation shifts from pleasing themselves and their partners to providing for their children. Therefore more resources (such as time and money) will be devoted to the children rather than the couple.

What else influences cheating behaviors? In an analysis of national data on sexual practice, Chien Liu found that the longer women are married, the less likely they are to cheat. This is partly based on the fact that women find more pleasure in the emotional aspects of a relationship than men. For men, however, the likelihood of cheating looks more like an upside down *U* shape, where men are more likely to cheat in the first 18 years of marriage (the chances of a man cheating increase every year) and then become less likely to cheat after 18 years of marriage (the chances of a man cheating decrease every year). Liu theorizes that because men have invested so much effort in the marriage, after 18 years, the benefits of marriage are greater, and the benefits of cheating (such as the excitement of sexual novelty) are not worth costing him his marriage.[21]

Denise Previti and Paul Amato investigated the role of marital satisfaction on the likelihood of one partner to cheat.[22] They found that in relationships where someone had not cheated but was in a relationship with a high likelihood of divorce, such as one partner thinking the marriage is in trouble or thinking or talking about divorce, it is likely that one person will engage in extramarital sex. They predicted and found that extramarital sex occurred more often in troubled marriages. Also, even if people are unhappy in their marriages, they are likely to cheat only after they start thinking and talking about divorce (with their partners or others). They hypothesized that people may cheat to try out new partners in anticipation of the marriage ending. They did not find any difference between how wives and husbands go through the process of deciding whether to cheat.

Paul Mongeau and Bobbi Schulz studied the verbal responses following sexual infidelity.[23] They most obvious possible response is that a person could lie and deny the cheating behaviors. Whether a person will lie and the degree to which the person will tell the truth is dependent on how much knowledge the accuser has. In other words, if someone is caught red-handed, then she will probably tell the truth. As Mongeau and Schulz wrote, "it is clear from the present data that the verbal responses presented following a transgression contained accounts, that is explanations for a rule violation, only when the partner already knew about the transgression."[24]

According to the study, if the cheater does tell the truth, he usually uses one of four explanations. The explanations involve concessions, excuses, justification, or refusals. The authors describe each of them as follows: concessions involve an admission of responsibility, an admission of feeling guilty, and/or an apology. In an excuse, the cheater admits that the rule violation occurred, however, she asserts that she had no way of controlling it. In justifications, the cheater takes responsibility for her actions, however, she denies that her actions were wrong, serious, or unwarranted. In a refusal, the cheater does not recognize his partner's right to request an account, asserting that the incident never occurred and/or that he does not need to provide an explanation for his behavior. Cheaters' de-

scriptions of the cheating were substantially more truthful as the partners' knowledge increased. Only when participants were sure that their
partners knew that they cheated did they mention the intimate details
of the infidelity. So it is likely that a cheater will lie about an incident if
the accuser does not have knowledge about the affair.

THE ROLE OF COMMUNICATION
BEHAVIORS IN SAVING A RELATIONSHIP:
RELATIONSHIP MAINTENANCE

In a study of communication episodes in unhealthy relationships, researchers found that dysfunctional, repetitive communication patterns are
extremely bad for relationships. Couples who fell into these patterns reported lack of communication satisfaction, avoidance of interaction, and
perceived unethical communication in the form of lies and game playing
with their partners. The researcher provided examples of what the couples said about their spouses. Comments included statements like "he
wouldn't listen," "our discussions always ended in an argument," "for
12 years, our only topic of conversation was the children," "all we ever
talked about was his job and his problems," or "I learned about a time she
was not honest with me."[25]

There were also communication episodes that involved couples arguing over a third party. These people were often perceived as a threat to
the couple by one of the partners. Comments from people in the study
included the following: "he was constantly belittling me in front of my
family and friends" and "I told one of our mutual friends how I felt and
she took it upon herself to tell my girlfriend."[26]

The hard truth is that relationships need maintenance, and it takes
a great deal of effort to sustain a romantic relationship. Dan Canary and
Laura Stafford "define relational maintenance behaviors as actions and
activities used to sustain desired relational qualities. This definition implies that people strategically engage in behaviors for the purposes of
sustaining important characteristics that are fundamental to intimate relationships. Such characteristics include features such as liking the partner, control mutuality (i.e., the extent to which partners agree on who
has the rightful influence power in various domains of decision making),
trust, commitment, and satisfaction."[27] Behaviors used to maintain a relationship must be continuous. They cannot be an effort that lasts a few
days or something done once. Canary and colleagues have found that

certain behaviors are used by people to sustain a relationship. These involve positivity, where people try to act nice and are cheerful and attempt to make shared activities enjoyable for both parties. There is openness, where one partner encourages the other to share thoughts and feelings and discuss the nature of the relationship. Providing a partner assurance is also essential; a person can remind someone of the commitment he made, that he is vested in a shared future, and that he is faithful. Also, sharing a social network is important. A person should be willing to spend time with the friends and family of a significant other and build common friends and affiliations. Two other important related maintenance features are sharing tasks and participating in joint activities. A person should do her fair share of household work and help equally to complete the tasks that need to be done. Couples also use mediated communication, such as the phone, texting, and e-mail, to communicate and maintain the relationship.[28] People are more likely to maintain relationships that are both equitable and rewarding.[29] Canary and other researchers often look at how household chores are completed and a general division of household labor because they believe it can accurately assess equity issues and how relationships and gender roles are maintained through interaction. Some of the maintenance strategies are unplanned and routine behaviors in which couples regularly engage, even when they are not making an effort to work on their relationship. Others are planned with the specific goal of enhancing the relationship. There are differences between maintenance strategies that are preemptive, in that they occur before major problems in the relationship, and those that are reactive, occurring after there have been problems or separation. We know neglect is destructive to relationships. Other ways to sustain a relationship are through encouraging mutual self-disclosure between couples, communicating acceptance and respect for a partner, and acknowledging the ways that each partner makes significant contributions to the relationship.[30]

COMMUNICATION THAT YOU SHOULD AVOID: ANGRY WITHDRAWAL, CONFLICT AVOIDANCE, AND INTIMACY AVOIDANCE

When a person or a partner starts to engage in withdrawal behaviors, it is time to have serious conversations about the relationship.[31] Nonverbal communication typical of withdrawal behavior is silence, lack of eye contact, and lack of affectionate touching. Verbal communications such as making a joke or changing the subject when relationship issues or sex come up are also withdrawal behaviors. Clearly these have different interpersonal meanings, depending on the situation and the topic. For example, if something is said during a fight, it would have a different meaning if it were said during a tender moment.

There are also healthy and unhealthy conflict styles and ways to remove oneself from the conflict. Canary and colleagues differentiated between offensive or stonewalling conflict disengagement style from a style that is defensive or distracting. Similarly, Canary believes it important to differentiate between angry withdrawal and conflict avoidance. Angry withdrawal results in more indirect communication involving displays of anger, hostility, rejection, or a combination of these emotions. People engaged in an angry withdrawal would be likely to stomp out of the room, pout, or give the silent treatment.

Conflict avoidance involves withdrawal from the conflict without a direct rejection of the partner and indirect communication of anger and hostility. Typical conflict avoidance behaviors include a change in the subject, making a joke, placating, failing to bring up a disagreement, or demonstrating a lack of interest or involvement in the discussion of a disagreement. Canary found that angry withdrawal is more related to marital distress than conflict avoidance. Perhaps this is because angry withdrawal is seen as functionally similar to overtly hostile acts by the partner. This could also be due to the fact that some researchers have suggested that for some couples, conflict avoidance may be a stable and functional adaptation to deal with conflict. Dr. Gottman, however, would disagree and believes that conflict avoidance is dysfunctional for couples because it leads to unresolved issues. Because couples are unique, conflict avoidance probably works for some couples and not for others. It is also concerning when one partner withdrawals from caregiving. If a partner starts to avoid intimacy and stops responding to a partner's needs for care and closeness, it is time to seriously worry about the relationship.

CONCLUSION

Many people believe that all societal ills could be cured with more communication or the right kind of communication. One thing is certain; communication is not a panacea or cure-all for relational and sexual problems. Relationships end; not everyone is going to stay together forever. Relationships deteriorate for many reasons, as many reasons as there are couples. Theoretically, each couple is unique, and reasons for relationship deterioration are unique to that couple. Realistically, there are some general causes to relational deterioration that are applicable to many breakups that researchers have identified and studied. Upon reflection of the research presented in this book, it is easy to identify some reasons that people get into relationships. One can see that relationships end when the relationships no longer meet one or both of the couples' needs. For example, one of the main reasons to be in a romantic relationship is to lessen loneliness. When being in the relationship no longer fulfils this need and one or both of the people feel lonely in the relationship, then the relationship may decay. Relationships also begin to provide stimulation, provide gains in knowledge and esteem, improve physical and mental health, and maximize pleasure and minimize pain.[32] When relationships fail to do these things, then they will dissolve. Clearly, even when marital relationships are impaired or diminished, external pressures may operate to keep partners in an unhealthy relationship. These external pressures include religious convictions; emotional costs to self and others; disapproval and/or sanctions from social or kin networks; investments of time, energy, money, and so on; and absence of attractive alternatives outside of the relationship. Keep in mind that some relationships are unhealthy and they should dissolve. If one or both members are not getting their basic relational requirements met, if couples have tried to fix the relationship, or if someone has committed an unforgivable act (such as cheating), then the relationship should end.

NOTES

1. Pamela Regan, *The Dating Game*, 2nd ed. (Thousand Oaks, CA: Sage, 2008), 90.

2. Diane Felmlee, "Fatal Attraction," in *The Dark Side of Close Relationships*, ed. William R. Cupach and Brian H. Spitzberg (Mahwah, NJ: Lawrence Erlbaum Associates, 1998), 3.

3. Laura K. Guerrero, Angela G. La Valley, and Lisa Farinelli, "The Experience and Expression of Anger, Guilt, and Sadness in Marriage: An Equity Theory Explanation," *Journal of Social and Personal Relationships* 25 (2008).

4. Brian Spitzberg and William Cupach, eds., *The Dark Side of Close Relationships* (Mahwah, NJ: Lawrence Erlbaum Associates, 1998), xi.

5. Ibid.

6. Ibid.

7. Ibid., xv.

8. Ibid., xiv.

9. Ibid.

10. Ibid.

11. Ibid., xv.

12. Ibid., xvii.

13. Christine L. Carson and William R. Cupach, "Fueling the Flames of the Green-Eyed Monster: The Role of Ruminative Thought in Reaction to Romantic Jealousy," *Western Journal of Communication* 64 (2000): 309.

14. Ibid., 313, including a reference from Laura K. Guerrero and Peter A. Andersen, "Coping with the Green-eyed Monsert: Conceptualizing and Measuring Communicative Responses to Romantic Jealousy," *Western Journal of Communication* 59 (1995): 270–304.

15. Ibid., 315, including a reference from Guerro and Anderson 1995.

16. Ibid., 316.

17. Ibid., 324.

18. Mary Crawford and Joseph Unger, *Women and Gender: A Feminist Psychology* (New York: McGraw-Hill, 2000).

19. Helen Kaplan, *The New Sex Therapy: Active Treatment of Sexual Dysfunctions* (New York: Times Books, 1974).

20. Mick P. Couper, and Linda L. Stinson, "National Health and Social Life Survey: Completion of Self-Administered Questionnaires in a Sex Survey," *Journal of Sex Research* 36 (1999): 321–30.

21. Chien Liu, "A Theory of Marital Sexual Life," *Journal of Marriage and Family* 62, no. 2 (2000). On p. 372, Liu explains the DINS dilemma. Some researchers attribute the declining frequency of marital sex with marital duration to fatigue from work or to the fact that both husband and wife work full-time outside the home and therefore do not have the interest or time for marital sex. This effect is referred to as the *DINS dilemma* (double income, no sex). Now, in light of the findings of Liu's paper, this explanation becomes questionable. Compared to marital sex, extramarital sex is much more time consuming and costly in terms of search and concealment. If couples who work full-time have no time for marital sex, they will have even less time to engage in extramarital sex. However, the preceding analysis shows that the likelihood of extramarital sex increases later in a couple's marriage, implying that the DINS explanation is not supported by the analysis developed here. Thus this study rules out the DINS explanation.

22. Denise Previti and Paul R. Amato, "Is Infidelity a Cause or a Consequence of Poor Marital Quality?" *Journal of Social and Personal Relationships* 21 (2004): 227–28.

23. Paul A. Mongeau and Bobbi E. Schulz, "What He Doesn't Know Won't Hurt Him (or Me): Verbal Responses and Attributions Following Sexual Infidelity," *Communication Reports* 10, no. 2 (1997): 143.

24. Ibid., 149.

25. William R. Cupach and Sandra Metts, "Accounts of Relational Dissolution: A Comparison of Marital and Non-marital Relationships," *Communication Monographs* 53 (1986): 321.

26. Ibid., 321.

27. Daniel J. Canary and Laura Stafford, "Equity in the Preservation of Personal Relationships," in *Close Romantic Relationships*, ed. Amy Wenzel and John Harvey (Mahwah, NJ: Lawrence Erlbaum Associates, 2003), 360.

28. Ibid., 135.

29. Ibid., 144.

30. Cupach and Metts, "Accounts of Relational Dissolution," 313.

31. Linda Roberts, "Fire and Ice in Marital Communication: Hostile and Distancing Behaviors as Predictors of Marital Distress," *Journal of Marriage and Family* 62, no. 3 (2000): 703–4. Daniel Canary, William Cupach, and S. J. Messman, *Relationship Conflict: Conflict in Parent-Child, Friendship, and Romantic Relationships* (Thousand Oaks, CA: Sage, 1995).

32. Joseph Devito, *The Interpersonal Communication Book* (New York: Longman, 2001), 272–73.

Bibliography

Abbey, Antonia. "Misperceptions of Friendly Behavior as Sexual Interest: A Survey of Naturally Occurring Incidents." *Psychology of Women Quarterly* 11, no. 2 (1987): 173–94.

Abbey, Antonia, Lisa Thompson Ross, Donna McDuffie, and Pam McAuslan. "Alcohol and Dating Risk Factors for Sexual Assault among College Women." *Psychology of Women Quarterly* 20, no. 1 (1996): 147–69.

Abrahams, Matthew F. "Perceiving Flirtatious Communication: An Exploration of the Perceptual Dimensions Underlying Judgments of Flirtatiousness." *Journal of Sex Research* 31 (1994): 283–92.

Afifi, Walid, and Alysa Lucas. "Information Seeking in the Initial Stages of Relational Development." In *Handbook of Relationship Initiation*, edited by Susan Sprecher, Amy Wenzel, and John Harvey, 135–51. New York: Psychology Press, 2008.

Allen, Mike, Tara Emmers-Sommer, and Tara Crowell. "Couples Negotiating Safer Sex Behaviors: A Meta-Analysis of the Impact of Conversation and Gender." In *Interpersonal Communication Research: Advances through Meta-Analysis*, edited by Raymond W. Preiss, Barbara Mae Gayle, and Nancy A. Burrell, 263–79. Mahwah, NJ: Lawrence Erlbaum Associates, 2002.

Andersen, Peter. *Nonverbal Communication: Forms and Function.* Mountain View, CA: Mayfield, 1999.

Aubrey, Jennifer Stevens. "Sex and Punishment: An Examination of Sexual Consequences and the Sexual Double Standard in Teen Programming." *Sex Roles* 50, no. 7 (2004): 505–14.

Bachmann, G.A., S.R. Leiblum, and J. Grill. "Brief Sexual Inquiry in Gynecologic Practice." *Obstetrics and Gynecology* 73, no. 3 Pt. 1 (1989): 425–27.

Bandura, Albert. *Social Foundations of Thought and Action: A Social Cognitive Theory.* Englewood Cliffs, NJ: Prentice Hall, 1986.

Baron, Robert A. "Sexual Arousal and Physical Aggression: The Inhibiting Influence of 'Cheesecake' and Nudes." *Bulletin of the Psychonomic Society* 3,
no. 5 (1974): 337–39.

Barratt, M. S., and W. L. Risser. "Sexual Terminology: A Barrier to Communication between Adolescents and Health Care Providers." *Ambulatory
Child Health* 4, no. 1 (1998): 21–31.

Bartky, Sandra Lee. *Femininity and Domination.* New York: Routledge, 1990.

Baumeister, Roy F. "Gender Differences in Erotic Plasticity: The Female Sex
Drive as Socially Flexible and Responsive." *Psychological Bulletin* 126,
no. 3 (2000): 347–74.

Baxter, Leslie A., and William W. Wilmot. "Secret Tests: Social Strategies for
Acquiring Information about the State of the Relationship." *Human Communication Research* 11 (1984): 171–202.

Bednarski, P. J. "Oh, Is TV Naughty." *Broadcasting and Cable* 133, no. 39
(2003): 37.

Bell, Robert A., and Nancy L. Buerkel-Rothfuss. "S(He) Loves Me, S(He)
Loves Me Not: Predictors of Relational Information-Seeking in Courtship and Beyond." *Communication Quarterly* 38 (1990): 64–82.

Berkowitz, Bob, and Susan Yaeger-Berkowitz. *He's Just Not up for It Anymore:
Why Men Stop Having Sex and What You Can Do about It.* New York: HarperCollins, 2007.

Blumstein, Philip, and Pepper Schwartz. *American Couples: Money, Work, Sex.*
New York: Morrow, 1983.

Boekeloo, B. O., L. A. Schamus, T. L. Cheng, and S. J. Simmens. "Young Adolescents' Comfort with Discussion about Sexual Problems with Their
Physician." *Archives of Pediatrics and Adolescent Medicine* 150, no. 11 (1996):
1146–52.

Bragg, Sarah, and David Buckingham. *Young People, Sex and the Media.* Hampshire, UK: Palgrave Macmillan, 2004.

Brown, Jane D. "Mass Media Influences on Sexuality." *Journal of Sex Research*
39 (2002): 42–45.

Burgoon, Judee. "Nonverbal Violations of Expectations." In *Nonverbal Interaction,* edited by J. M. Wiemann and R. P. Harrison, 77–111. Beverly Hills,
CA: Sage, 1983.

Burgoon, Judee, Joseph Walther, and James Baesler. "Interpretations, Evaluations, and Consequences of Interpersonal Touch." *Human Communication Research* 19, no. 2 (1992): 237–63.

Bussey, Kay, and Albert Bandura. "Social Cognitive Theory of Gender Development and Differentiation." *Psychological Review* 106, no. 4 (1999):
676–713.

Canary, Daniel, William Cupach, and S. J. Messman. *Relationship Conflict: Conflict in Parent-Child, Friendship, and Romantic Relationships.* Thousand Oaks,
CA: Sage, 1995.

Canary, Daniel J., Brian H. Spitzberg, Beth A. Semic, Peter A. Andersen, and
Laura K. Guerrero. "The Experience and Expression of Anger in Inter-

personal Settings." In *Handbook of Communication and Emotion: Research, Theory, Applications, and Contexts*, 189–213. San Diego, CA: Academic Press, 1998.

Canary, Daniel J., and Laura Stafford. "Equity in the Preservation of Personal Relationships." In *Close Romantic Relationships*, edited by Amy Wenzel and John Harvey, 133–51. Mahwah, NJ: Lawrence Erlbaum Associates, 2003.

Cancian, Francesca. "Love and the Rise of Capitalism." In *Gender in Intimate Relationships: A Micro Structural Approach*, edited by Barbara Riseman and Pepper Schwartz, 12–25. Belmont, CA: Wadsworth, 1989.

Carl, Walter J., and Steve Duck. "How to Do Things with Relationships . . . and How Relationships Do Things with Us." In *Communication Year-book*, edited by Pamela Kalbfleisch, 1–37. Mahwah, NJ: Lawrence Erlbaum Associates, 2004.

Carson, Christine L., and William R. Cupach. "Fueling the Flames of the Green-Eyed Monster: The Role of Ruminative Thought in Reaction to Romantic Jealousy." *Western Journal of Communication* 64 (2000): 308–30.

Caruthers, Allison S. "'Hookups' and 'Friends with Benefits': Nonrelational Sexual Encounters as Contexts of Women's Normative Sexual Development," University of Michigan, ProQuest Information & Learning, 2006.

Catania, J. A., T. J. Coates, R. Stall, H. Turner, J. Peterson, N. Hearst, M. M. Dolcini, et al. "Prevalence of AIDS-Related Risk Factors and Condom Use in the United States." *Science* 258, no. 5085 (1992): 1101–6.

Centers for Disease Control and Prevention. "Adolescent Reproductive Health: Research." Centers for Disease Control and Prevention. http://www.cdc.gov.

Centers for Disease Control and Prevention. "HIV/AIDS Surveillance Report: Cases of HIV Infection and AIDS in the United States, 2005." Centers for Disease Control and Prevention. http://www.cdc.gov/hiv/stats/2005SurveillanceReport.pdf.

Centers for Disease Control and Prevention. "Pneumocystis Pneumonia—Los Angeles." In *Mortality and Morbidity Weekly Report 1981*, 250–52. Atlanta, GA: Centers for Disease Control and Prevention, 1981.

Check, James V., and Neil M. Malamuth. "Sex Role Stereotyping and Reactions to Depictions of Stranger versus Acquaintance Rape." *Journal of Personality and Social Psychology* 45, no. 2 (1983): 344–56.

Chein, Liu. "Does Quality of Marital Sex Decline with Duration?" *Archives of Sexual Behavior* 32 (2003): 55–60.

Christopher, F. Scott, and Susan Sprecher. "Sexuality in Marriage, Dating, and Other Relationships: A Decade Review." *Journal of Marriage and Family* 62, no. 4 (2000): 999–1017.

Chu, Amy. "Teen Movies as Sex Education Material? A Content Analysis of Popular Teen Movies in Four Decades." Paper presented at the annual meeting of the International Communication Association, San Francisco, 2007.

Clawson, Carolyn, and Marla Reese-Weber. "The Amount and Timing of Parent-Adolescent Sexual Communication as Predictors of Late Adolescent Sexual Risk-Taking Behaviors." *Journal of Sex Research* 40 (2003): 256–65.

Cleary, Jennifer, Richard Barhman, Terry MacCormack, and Ed Herold. "Discussing Sexual Health with a Partner: A Qualitative Study with Young Women." *Canadian Journal of Human Sexuality* 11 (2002): 117–33.

Cline, Rebecca Welch, K. Freeman, and S. Johnson. "Talk among Sexual Partners about AIDS: Interpersonal Communication for Risk Reduction or Risk Enhancement?" *Health Communication* 4 (1992): 39–56.

Cohen, L. L., and R. L. Shotland. "Timing of First Sexual Intercourse in a Relationship: Expectations, Experiences, and Perceptions of Others." *Journal of Sex Research* 33, no. 4 (1996): 291–99.

Coleman, L. M., and R. Ingham. "Exploring Young People's Difficulties in Talking about Contraception: How Can We Encourage More Discussion between Partners?" *Health Education Research* 14, no. 6 (1999): 741–50.

College of New Jersey, The. "*Today Show, Newsweek* Feature Research of TCNJ Professor." Press release. http://www.tcnj.edu/~pa/news/2004/BethPaul.htm.

Consumer Reports Health. "80% of Sexually Active Americans Put Off Sex Because They're Too Sick or Tired." *Consumer Reports*. http://pressroom.consumerreports.org/pressroom/2009/02/consumer-reports-health-poll-80-of-sexually-active-americans-put-off-sex-because-theyre-too-sick-or-.html.

Council on Scientific Affairs, American Medical Association. "Health Care Needs of Gay Men and Lesbians in the United States." *Journal of the American Medical Association* 275, no. 17 (1996): 1354–59.

Crawford, Mary, and Joseph Unger. *Women and Gender: A Feminist Psychology*. New York: McGraw-Hill, 2000.

Cunningham, Michael, and Anita Barbee. "Prelude to a Kiss: Nonverbal Flirting, Opening Gambits, and Other Communication Dynamics in the Initiation of Romantic Relationships." In *Handbook of Relationship Initiation*, edited by Susan Sprecher, Amy Wenzel, and John Harvey, 97–120. New York: Psychology Press, 2008.

Cupach, William R., and Sandra Metts. "Accounts of Relational Dissolution: A Comparison of Marital and Non-marital Relationships." *Communication Monographs* 53 (1986): 311–34.

Davison, Sonia L., Robin J. Bell, Maria LaChina, Samantha L. Holden, and Susan R. Davis. "Sexual Function in Well Women: Stratification by Sexual Satisfaction, Hormone Use, and Menopause Status." *Journal of Sexual Medicine* 5, no. 5 (2008): 1214–22.

Derlega, Valerian, Barbara Winstead, and Kathryn Greene. "Self-Disclosure and Starting a Close Relationship." In *Handbook of Relationship Initiation*, edited by Susan Sprecher, Amy Wenzel, and John Harvey, 153–74. New York: Psychology Press, 2008.

de Visser, Richard, Anthony Smith, Chris E. Rissel, Juliet Richters, and Andrew E. Grulich. "Sex in Australia: Safer Sex and Condom Use Among a Representative Sample of Adults." *Australian and New Zealand Journal of Public Health* 27, no. 12 (2007): 223–29.

Devito, Joseph. *The Interpersonal Communication Book*. New York: Longman, 2001.

DiCenso, A., V. W. Borthwick, C. A. Busca, C. Creatura, J. A. Holmes, W. F. Kalagian, and B. M. Partington. "Completing the Picture: Adolescents Talk about What's Missing in Sexual Health Services." *Canadian Journal of Public Health* 92, no. 1 (2001): 35–38.

diMauro, Diane. *Sexuality Research in the United States: An Assessment of the Social and Behavioral Sciences*. New York: Social Science Research Council, 1995.

Donnerstein, E., M. Donnerstein, and R. Evans. "Erotic Stimuli and Aggression: Facilitation or Inhibition." *Journal of Personality and Social Psychology* 32, no. 2 (1975): 237–44.

Downey, Jerrold L., and William F. Vitulli. "Self-Report Measures of Behavioral Attributions Related to Interpersonal Flirtation Situations." *Psychological Reports* 61, no. 3 (1987): 899–904.

Duck, Steve. "Where Do All the Kisses Go? Rapport, Positivity and Relational-Level Analyses of Interpersonal Enmeshment." *Psychological Inquiry* 1, no. 4 (1990): 308–9.

Duck, Steve, Linda West, and L. K. Acitelli. "Sewing the Field: The Tapestry of Relationships in Life and Research." In *Handbook of Personal Relationships*, edited by Steve Duck, 1–23. Chichester, NY: John Wiley, 1997.

Duck, Steve and Susan Sprecher. "Sweet Talk: The Importance of Perceived Communication for Romantic and Friendship Attraction Experienced During a Get-Acquainted Date." *Personality and Social Psychology Bulletin* 20, no. 4 (August 1994): 391–400.

Eastwick, Paul, and Eli Finkel. "Speed-Dating: A Powerful and Flexible Paradigm for Studying Romantic Relationship Initiation." In *Handbook of Relationship Initiation*, edited by Susan Sprecher, Amy Wenzel, and John Harvey, 217–34. New York: Psychology Press, 2008.

Edgar, Timothy, Vicki Friemuth, S. Hammond, D. McDonald, and Edgar Fink. "Strategic Sexual Communication: Condom Use Resistance and Response." *Health Communication* 4 (1992): 83–104.

Egland, Kori I., Brian H. Spitzberg, and Michelle M. Zormeier. "Flirtation and Conversational Competence in Cross-Sex Platonic and Romantic Relationships." *Communication Reports* 9 (1996): 105–17.

Eldridge, Kathleen A., Mia Sevier, Janice Jones, David C. Atkins, and Andrew Christensen. "Demand-Withdraw Communication in Severely Distressed, Moderately Distressed, and Nondistressed Couples: Rigidity and Polarity during Relationship and Personal Problem Discussions." *Journal of Family Psychology* 21 (2007): 218–26.

Elliott, Sinikka, and Debra Umberson. "The Performance of Desire: Gender and Sexual Negotiation in Long-Term Marriages." *Journal of Marriage and Family* 70, no. 2 (2008): 391–406.

Ellis, Bruce J., and Donald Symons. "Sex Differences in Sexual Fantasy: An Evolutionary Psychological Approach." *Journal of Sex Research* 27, no. 4 (1990): 527–55.

Emmers-Sommer, Tara M., and Mike Allen. "HIV and AIDS: Toward Increased Awareness and Understanding of Prevention and Education Research Using Meta-Analysis." *Communication Studies* 52, no. 2 (2001): 127–41.

England, Paula, and George Farkas. *Households, Employment, and Gender: A Social, Economic, and Demographic View.* Hawthorne, NY: Aldine, 1986.

Eyal, Keren, and Keli Finnerty. "The Portrayal of Sexual Intercourse on Television: How, Who, and with What Consequence?" *Mass Communication and Society* 12 (2009): 143–69.

Farris, Coreen, Teresa A. Treat, Richard J. Viken, and Richard M. McFall. "Perceptual Mechanisms That Characterize Gender Differences in Decoding Women's Sexual Intent." *Psychological Science* 19 (2008): 348–54.

Fehr, Beverley. "Friendship Formation." In *Handbook of Relationship Initiation*, edited by Susan Sprecher, Amy Wenzel, and John Harvey, 29–54. New York: Psychology Press, 2008.

Felmlee, Diane. "Fatal Attraction." In *The Dark Side of Close Relationships*, edited by William R. Cupach and Brian H. Spitzberg, 3–31. Mahwah, NJ: Lawrence Erlbaum Associates, 1998.

Fisher, Deborah A., Douglas L. Hill, Joel W. Grube, and Enid L. Gruber. "Sex on American Television: An Analysis across Program Genres and Network Types." *Journal of Broadcasting and Electronic Media* 48 (2004): 529–53.

Fisher, Helen. "Broken Hearts: The Nature and Risk of Romantic Rejection." In *Romance and Sex in Adolescence and Emerging Adulthood: Risks and Opportunities*, edited by Ann C. Crouter and Alan Booth, 3–28. Mahwah, NJ: Lawrence Erlbaum Associates, 2006.

Fisher, T. D. "Parent-Child Communication about Sex and Young Adolescents' Sexual Knowledge and Attitudes." *Adolescence* 21, no. 83 (1986): 517–27.

Floyd, Kory, and Sarah Riforgiate. "Affectionate Communication Received from Spouses Predicts Stress Hormone Levels in Healthy Adults." *Communication Monographs* 75, no. 4 (2008): 351–68.

Freedman, Jonathan. *Happy People: What Happiness Is, Who Has It and Why.* New York: Ballantine, 1978.

Furman, Wyndol, and Laura Shaffer Hand. "The Slippery Nature of Romantic Relationships: Issues in Definition and Differentiation." In *Romance and Sex in Adolescence and Emerging Adulthood: Risks and Opportunities*, edited by Ann C. Crouter and Alan Booth, 171–78. Mahwah, NJ: Lawrence Erlbaum Associates, 2006.

Gagnon, John, and William Simon. *Sexual Conduct: The Social Sources of Human Sexuality*. Chicago: Aldine-Atherton Press, 1973.

Gerbert, Barbara, Dale Danley, Dung Huynh, Daniel Ciccarone, Paul Gilbert, David Bangsberg, Kathleen Clanon, Anas Hana, and Michael Allerton. *Bet You and Your Doctor Don't Talk about Sex: A Conversation Starter for HIV-Positive Men and Women*. San Francisco: University of California Center for Health Improvement and Prevention Studies.

Gilbert, David, Yvonne Guerrier, and Jonathan Guy. "Sexual Harassment Issues in the Hospitality Industry." *International Journal of Contemporary Hospitality Management* 10 (1998): 48–53.

Ginsburg, G. P. "Rules, Scripts, and Prototypes in Personal Relationships." In *Handbook of Personal Relationships*, edited by Steven Duck, 23–39. London: John Wiley, 1988.

Giraldi, Anna Maria. "Sex Is Here to Stay." *Journal of Sex Medicine* 5 (2008): 2737–739.

Glenn, Norval, and Elizabeth Marquardt. *Hooking Up, Hanging Out and Hoping for Mr. Right: College Women on Dating and Mating Today*. New York: Institute of American Values, 2001.

Goffman, Irvin. *Interaction Rituals: Essays on Face to Face Behavior*. Garden City, NY: Doubleday, 1967.

Gonzaga, Gian, Dacher Keltner, Esme Londahl, and Michael Smith. "Love and the Commitment Problem in Romantic Relations and Friendship." *Journal of Personality and Social Psychology* 81, no. 2 (2001): 247–62.

Gray, John. *Men Are from Mars, Women Are from Venus*. New York: HarperCollins, 1992.

Graziano, William, and Jennifer Weisho Bruce. "Attraction and the Initiation of Relationships: A Review of the Empirical Literature." In *Handbook of Relationship Initiation*, edited by Susan Sprecher, Amy Wenzel, and John Harvey, 269–95. New York: Psychology Press, 2008.

Greenberg, Bradley, and Rick Busselle. *Soap Operas and Sexual Activity*. Menlo Park, CA: Kaiser Family Foundation, 1994.

Greenberg, Bradley, C. Stanley, M. Siemicki, C. Heeter, A. Soderman, and R. Linsangan. "Sex Content on Soaps and Prime-Time Television Series Most Viewed by Adolescents." In *Media, Sex, and the Adolescent*, edited by Bradely Greenberg, Jane Brown, and Nancy Buerkel-Rothfuss, 29–44. Cresskill, NJ: Hampton, 1993.

Greene, Kathryn, and Sandra Faulkner. "Gender, Belief in the Sexual Double Standard, and Sexual Talk in Heterosexual Dating Relationships." *Sex Roles* 53 (2005): 239–51.

Gueguen, Nicolas, and Jacques Fischer-Lokou. "Another Evaluation of Touch and Helping Behavior." *Psychological Reports* 92, no. 1 (2003): 62–64.

Guerrero, Laura, and Peter Andersen. "Coping with the Green-eyed Monster: Conceptualizing and Measuring Communicative Responses to Romantic Jealousy." *Western Journal of Communication* 59 (1995): 270–304.

Guerrero, Laura K., and Peter A. Andersen. "The Waxing and Waning of Relational Intimacy: Touch as a Function of Relational Stage, Gender and Touch Avoidance." *Journal of Social and Personal Relationships* 8, no. 2 (1991): 147–65.

Guerrero, Laura K., Susanne M. Jones, and Judee K. Burgoon. "Responses to Nonverbal Intimacy Change in Romantic Dyads: Effects of Behavioral Valence and Degree of Behavioral Change on Nonverbal and Verbal Reactions." *Communication Monograph* 67, no. 4 (2000): 325–46.

Guerrero, Laura K., Angela G. La Valley, and Lisa Farinelli. "The Experience and Expression of Anger, Guilt, and Sadness in Marriage: An Equity Theory Explanation." *Journal of Social and Personal Relationships* 25 (2008): 699–724.

Guerrero, Laura, and Paul Mongeau. "On Becoming 'More Than Friends': The Transition from Friendship to Romantic Relationship." In *Handbook of Relationship Initiation*, edited by Susan Sprecher, Amy Wenzel, and John Harvey, 175–94. New York: Psychology Press, 2008.

Guzman, Bianca L., Michelle Schlehofer-Sutton, and Christina M. Villanueva. "Let's Talk about Sex: How Comfortable Discussions about Sex Impact Teen Sexual Behavior." *Journal of Health Communication* 8 (2003): 583–98.

Haboubi, N.H.J., and N. Lincoln. "Views of Health Professionals on Discussing Sexual Issues with Patients." *Disability and Rehabilitation* 25, no. 6 (2003): 291–96.

Haglund, K. "Recommendations for Sexuality Education for Early Adolescents." *Journal of Obstetric, Gynecologic, and Neonatal Nursing* 35, no. 3 (2006): 369–75.

Halford, Kim, Matthew Sanders, and Brett Behrens. "Can Skills Training Prevent Relationship Problems in at-Risk Couples? Four-Year Effects of a Behavioral Relationship Education Program." *Journal of Family Psychology* 15 (2001): 750–68.

Hall, Edward. *The Silent Language*. Garden City, NY: Anchor Press, 1973.

Hall, Jeffrey, Michael Cody, Grace Jackson, and Jacqueline Flesh. "Beauty and the Flirt: Attractiveness and Approaches to Relationship Initiation." In *International Communication Association*, 1–49. Montreal: International Communication Association, 2008.

Haselton, Martie G., and Daniel Nettle. "The Paranoid Optimist: An Integrative Evolutionary Model of Cognitive Biases." *Personality and Social Psychology Review* 10, no. 1 (2006): 47–66.

Hecht, Michael, Joseph DeVito, and Laura Guerrero. "Perspectives on Nonverbal Communication: Codes, Functions, and Contexts." In *The Nonverbal Communication Reader: Classic and Contemporary Readings*, edited by Laura Guerrero, Joseph DeVito, and Michael Hecht, 3–18. Prospect Heights, IL: Waveland Press, 1999.

Heisler, Jennifer M. "Family Communication about Sex: Parents and College-Aged Offspring Recall Discussion Topics, Satisfaction, and Parental Involvement." *Journal of Family Communication* 5 (2005): 295–312.

Helman, Cecil. *Culture, Health and Illness.* 2nd ed. London: Wright, 1990.

Henningsen, David Dryden. "Flirting with Meaning: An Examination of Miscommunication in Flirting Interactions." *Sex Roles* 50, no. 7 (2004): 481–89.

Henningsen, David Dryden, Mary Braz, and Elaine Davies. "Why Do We Flirt?" *Journal of Business Communication* 45 (2008): 483–502.

Henningsen, David Dryden, Mary Lynn Miller Henningsen, and Kathleen S. Valde. "Gender Differences in Perceptions of Women's Sexual Interest during Cross-Sex Interactions: An Application and Extension of Cognitive Valence Theory." *Sex Roles* 54, no. 11 (2006): 821–29.

Herold, Edward, Eleanor Maticka-Tyndale, and Dawn Mewhinney. "Predicting Intentions to Engage in Casual Sex." *Journal of Social and Personal Relationships* 15 (1998): 502–16.

Heslin, Richard, Tuan D. Nguyen, and Michele L. Nguyen. "Meaning of Touch: The Case of Touch from a Stranger or Same Sex Person." *Journal of Nonverbal Behavior* 7, no. 3 (1983): 147–57.

Hetsroni, Amir. "Overrepresented Topics, Underrepresented Topics, and the Cultivation Effect." *Communication Research Reports* 25 (2008): 200–10.

Hoff, Tina, Andrea Miller, Jennifer Barefoot, and Liberty Greene. "National Survey of Women about Their Sexual Health: Take Charge of Your Sexual Health." Kaiser Family Foundation. http://www.kff.org/womens health/20030618a-index.cfm.

Holmberg, Diane, and Samantha MacKenzie. "So Far, So Good: Scripts for Romantic Relationship Development as Predictors of Relational Well-Being." *Journal of Social and Personal Relationships* 19 (2002): 777–96.

Hordern, A.J., and A.F. Street. "Let's Talk about Sex: Risky Business for Cancer and Palliative Care Clinicians." *Contemporary Nurse* 27, no. 1 (2007): 49–60.

Hughes, Mikayla, Kelly Morrison, and Kelli Jean K. Asada. "What's Love Got to Do with It? Exploring the Impact of Maintenance Rules, Love Attitudes, and Network Support on Friends with Benefits Relationships." *Western Journal of Communication* 69 (2005): 49–66.

Hyde, Janet Shibley. "The Gender Similarities Hypothesis." *American Psychologist* 60, no. 6 (2005): 581–92.

Hyde, Janet Shibley, and John D. DeLamater. *Understanding Human Sexuality.* 7th ed. New York: McGraw-Hill, 2000.

Impett, Emily, Amy Strachman, Eli Finkel, and Shelly Gable. "Maintaining Sexual Desire in Intimate Relationships: The Importance of Approach Goals." *Journal of Personality and Social Psychology* 94, no. 5 (2008): 808–23.

Ivy, Diana, and Phil Backlund. *Genderspeak: Personal Effectiveness in Gender Communication.* Boston: McGraw-Hill, 2004.

Jackson, Susan, and Fiona Cram. "Disrupting the Sexual Double Standard: Young Women's Talk about Heterosexuality." *British Journal of Social Psychology* 42, Pt. 1 (2003): 113–27.

James, Susan Donaldson. "Study Reports Anal Sex on Rise among Teens: Lack of Sex Education, Virginity Pledges, Ignorance Contribute to Risky Behavior." ABC News, http://abcnews.go.com/Health/story?id=64280 03&page=1.

Jones, Stanley E., and Elaine Yarbrough. "A Naturalistic Study of the Meanings of Touch." *Communication Monographs* 52, no. 1 (1985): 19–56.

Judd, Ben B., Jr., and M. Wayne Alexander. "On the Reduced Effectiveness of Some Sexually Suggestive Ads." *Journal of the Academy of Marketing Science* 11, no. 2 (1983): 156–69.

Kann, Laura. "The Youth Risk Behavior Surveillance System: Measuring Health-Risk Behaviors." *American Journal of Health Behavior* 25, no. 3 (2001): 272–77.

Kantor, L. M. "Scared Chaste? Fear-Based Educational Curricula." *SIECUS Report* 21, no. 2 (1993): 1–15.

Kaplan, Helen. *The New Sex Therapy: Active Treatment of Sexual Dysfunctions.* New York: Times Books, 1974.

Kenrick, Douglas T., Edward K. Sadalla, Gary Groth, and Melanie R. Trost. "Evolution, Traits, and the Stages of Human Courtship: Qualifying the Parental Investment Model." *Journal of Personality* 58 (1990): 97–116.

Kimmel, Michael, and Jeffrey Fracher. "Hard Issues and Soft Spots: Counseling Men about Sexuality." In *Men's Lives,* edited by Michael Kimmel and Michael Messner, 438–50. New York: Macmillan, 1992.

Kinsey, Alfred, Wardell Pomeroy, and Clyde Martin. *Sexual Behavior in the Human Male.* Philadelphia: W. B. Saunders, 1948.

Kinsey, Alfred C., Wardell B. Pomeroy, Clyde E. Martin, and Paul H. Gebhard. *Sexual Behavior in the Human Female.* Oxford: W. B. Saunders, 1953.

Knapp, Mark, and Judith Hall. *Nonverbal Communication in Human Interaction.* 5th ed. Belmont, CA: Wadsworth/Thomson Learning, 2002.

Knobloch, Leanne K., and Katy E. Carpenter-Theune. "Topic Avoidance in Developing Romantic Relationships." *Communication Research* 31 (2004): 173–205.

Koeppel, Liana, Yvette Montagne-Miller, Dan O'Hair, and Michael Cody. "Friendly? Flirting? Wrong?" In *Interpersonal Communication: Evolving Interpersonal Relationships,* edited by Pamela Kalbfleisch, 13–32. Hillsdale, NJ: Lawrence Erlbaum Associates, 1993.

Koerner, Ascan F., and Mary Anne Fitzpatrick. "Nonverbal Communication and Marital Adjustment and Satisfaction: The Role of Decoding Relationship Relevant and Relationship Irrelevant Affect." *Communication Monographs* 69, no. 1 (2002): 33–52.

Koerner, Ascan F., and Mary Anne Fitzpatrick. "Toward a Theory of Family Communication." *Communication Theory* 12 (2002): 70–92.

Koesten, Joy. "Family Communication Patterns, Sex of Subject, and Communication Competence." *Communication Monographs* 71 (2004): 226–44.

Korobov, Neill, and Avril Thorne. "How Late-Adolescent Friends Share Stories about Relationships: The Importance of Mitigating the Seriousness of Romantic Problems." *Journal of Social and Personal Relationships* 24 (2007): 971–92.

Kraut-Becher, Julie, and Sevgi Aral. "Gap Length: An Important Factor in Sexually Transmitted Disease Transmission." *Sexually Transmitted Diseases* 30 (2003): 221–26.

Kuhn, D. "Intimacy, Sexuality, and Residents with Dementia." *Alzheimer's Care Quarterly* 3, no. 2 (2002): 165–73.

Kunkel, Dale, Kirstie Cope, Wendy Jo Farinola, Emma Rollin, and Edward Donnerstein. "Sex on TV: A Biennial Report to the Kaiser Family Foundation." Menlo Park, CA: Kaiser Family Foundation, 1999.

Kunkel, Dale, Kirstie Cope-Farrar, Erica Biely, Wendy Jo Farinola, and Edward Donnerstein. "Sex on TV, 2: A Biennial Report to the Kaiser Family Foundation." Menlo Park, CA: Kaiser Family Foundation, 2001.

Kunkel, Dale, Keren Eyal, Keli Finnerty, Erica Biely, and Edward Donnerstein. "Sex on TV, 4." Menlo Park, CA: Kaiser Family Foundation, 2005.

Lambert, Tracy A., Arnold S. Kahn, and Kevin J. Apple. "Pluralistic Ignorance and Hooking Up." *Journal of Sex Research* 40, no. 2 (2003): 129–33.

Langloise, Judith, and L. Roggman. "Attractive Faces Are Only Average." *Psychological Science* 1 (1990): 115–21.

LaPlante, Marcia N., Naomi McCormick, and Gary G. Brannigan. "Living the Sexual Script: College Students' Views of Influence in Sexual Encounters." *Journal of Sex Research* 16, no. 4 (1980): 338–55.

Laroche, Christiane, and Gaston-Rene de Grace. "Factors of Satisfaction Associated with Happiness in Adults." *Canadian Journal of Counselling* 31, no. 4 (1997): 275–86.

Laumann, Edward, Anthony Paik, Dale B. Glasser, Jeong-Han Kang, Tianfu Wang, Bernard Levinson, Edson Moreira, Alfredo Nicolosi, and Clive Gingel. "The Pfizer Global Study of Sexual Attitudes and Behaviors." Pfizer. http://www.pfizerglobalstudy.com/study/study-results.asp.

Laumann, Edward, John Gagnon, Robert Michael, S. Michaels, M. P. Couper, and L. L. Stinson. "National Health and Social Life Survey: Completion of Self-Administered Questionnaires in a Sex Survey." *Journal of Sex Research* 36 (1999): 321–30.

Laumann, Edward, Robert Michael, and John Gagnon. "A Political History of the National Sex Survey of Adults." *Family Planning Perspectives* 26, no. 1 (1994): 34–38.

Lefkowitz, Eva S., and Graciela Espinosa-Hernandez. "Sex-Related Communication with Mothers and Close Friends during the Transition to University." *Journal of Sex Research* 44 (2007): 17–27.

Le Poire, Beth A., and Judee K. Burgoon. "Two Contrasting Explanations of Involvement Violations: Expectancy Violations Theory versus Discrepancy Arousal Theory." *Human Communication Research* 20 (1994): 560–91.

Levant, Ronald F., and Katherine Richmond. "A Review of Research on Masculinity Ideologies Using the Male Role Norms Inventory." *Journal of Men's Studies* 15 (2007): 130–46.

Levine, Elana. *Wallowing in Sex: The New Sexual Culture of 1970s American Television.* Durham, NC: Duke University Press, 2007.

Levine, Timothy R., Krystyna Strzyzewski Aune, and Hee Sun Park. "Love Styles and Communication in Relationships: Partner Preferences, Initiation, and Intensification." *Communication Quarterly* 54 (2006): 465–86.

Lindau, Stacy, Natalia Gavrilova, and David Anderson. "Sexual Morbidity in Very Long Term Survivors of Vaginal and Cervical Cancer: A Comparison to National Norms." *Gynecologic Oncology* 106, no. 2 (2007): 413–18.

Lindau, Stacy Tessler, L. Philip Schumm, Edward O. Laumann, Wendy Levinson, Colm A. O'Muircheartaigh, and Linda J. Waite. "A Study of Sexuality and Health among Older Adults in the United States." *New England Journal of Medicine* 357, no. 8 (2007): 762–74.

Lisak, David. http://SPSMM@Lists.apa.org (Accessed July 6, 2006).

Liu, Chien. "A Theory of Marital Sexual Life." *Journal of Marriage and Family* 62, no. 2 (2000): 363–74.

Lorber, Judith. *Gender Inequality: Feminist Theories and Politics.* 2nd ed. Los Angeles, CA: Roxbury Press, 2001.

Lowry, Dennis T., and Jon A. Shidler. "Prime Time TV Portrayals of Sex, 'Safe Sex' and AIDS: A Longitudinal Analysis." *Journalism Quarterly* 70, no. 3 (1993): 628–37.

MacNeil, Sheila, and E. Sandra Byers. "The Relationships between Sexual Problems, Communication, and Sexual Satisfaction." *Canadian Journal of Human Sexuality* 6, no. 4 (1997): 277–83.

Magnan, M. A., and K. Reynolds. "Barriers to Addressing Patient Sexuality Concerns across Five Areas of Specialization." *Clinical Nurse Specialist* 20, no. 6 (2006): 285–92.

Manning, Wendy D., Peggy C. Giordano, and Monica A. Longmore. "Hooking Up: The Relationship Contexts of 'Nonrelationship' Sex." *Journal of Adolescent Research* 21, no. 5 (2006): 459–83.

Marks, Michael J., and R. Chris Fraley. "The Sexual Double Standard: Fact or Fiction?" *Sex Roles* 52 (2005): 175–86.

Marwick, Charles. "Survey Says Patients Expect Little Physician Help on Sex." *Journal of the American Medical Association* 281 (1999): 2173–74.

McGee, Elizabeth, and Mark Shevlin. "Effect of Humor on Interpersonal Attraction and Mate Selection." *Journal of Psychology* 143 (2009): 67–77.

McKay, Alexander, and Philippa Holowaty. "Sexual Health Education: A Study of Adolescents' Opinions, Self-Perceived Needs, and Current and Preferred Sources of Information." *Canadian Journal of Human Sexuality* 6, no. 1 (1997): 29–38.

McKenna, Katelyn. "MySpace or Your Place: Relationship Initiation and Development of the Wired and Wireless World." In *Handbook of Relationship Initiation*, edited by Susan Sprecher, Amy Wenzel, and John Harvey, 235–47. New York: Psychology Press, 2008.

McNulty, James K., and Terri D. Fisher. "Gender Differences in Response to Sexual Expectancies and Changes in Sexual Frequency: A Short-Term Longitudinal Study of Sexual Satisfaction in Newly Married Couples." *Archives of Sexual Behavior* 37 (2008): 229–40.

Metts, Sandra, and William R. Cupach. "The Role of Communication in Human Sexuality." In *Human Sexuality: The Societal and Interpersonal Context*, edited by Kathleen McKinney and Susan Sprecher, 139–61. Westport, CT: Ablex, 1989.

Metts, Sandra, and Sylvia Mikucki. "The Emotional Landscape of Romantic Relationship Initiation." In *Handbook of Relationship Initiation*, edited by Susan Sprecher, Amy Wenzel, and John Harvey, 353–71. New York: Psychology Press, 2008.

Metts, Sandra, and Brian Spitzberg. "Sexual Communication in Interpersonal Contexts: A Script-Based Approach." In *Communication Yearbook*, edited by Brant Burleson, 49–91. Mahwah, NJ: Lawrence Erlbaum Associates, 1996.

Michael, Robert. "Private Sex and Public Policy." In *Sex, Love, and Health in America: Private Choices and Public Policies*, edited by Edward Laumann and Robert Michael, 465–92. Chicago: University of Chicago Press, 2000.

Michael, Robert T., John H. Gagnon, Edward O. Laumann, and Gina Kolata. *Sex in America: A Definitive Survey.* Boston: Little, Brown, 1995.

Michels, Tricia M., Rhonda Y. Kropp, Stephen L. Eyre, and Bonnie L. Halpern-Felsher. "Initiating Sexual Experiences: How Do Young Adolescents Make Decisions Regarding Early Sexual Activity?" *Journal of Research on Adolescence* 15, no. 4 (2005): 583–607.

Middleton, DeWight. *Exotics and Erotics: Human Cultural and Sexual Diversity.* Prospect Heights, IL: Waveland, 2002.

Middleton, Robert, and Edward Laumann. "Introduction: Setting the Scene." In *Sex, Love, and Health in America: Private Choices and Public Policies*, edited by Robert Middleton and Edward Laumann, 1–38. Chicago: University of Chicago Press, 2002.

Milhausen, Robin, and Edward Herold. "Does the Sexual Double Standard Still Exist? Perceptions of University Women." *Journal of Sex Research* 36 (1999): 361–68.

Milhausen, Robin, and Edward Herold. "Reconceptualizing the Sexual Double Standard." *Journal of Psychology and Human Sexuality* 13, no. 63–83 (2001): 63–83.

Mongeau, Paul A., and Bobbi E. Schulz. "What He Doesn't Know Won't Hurt Him (or Me): Verbal Responses and Attributions Following Sexual Infidelity." *Communication Reports* 10, no. 2 (1997): 143–52.

Mongeau, Paul A., Janet Jacobsen, and Carolyn Donnerstein. "Defining Dates and First Date Goals: Generalizing from Undergraduates to Single Adults." *Communication Research* 34 (2007): 526–47.

Mongeau, Paul, and Colleen Carey. "Who's Wooing Whom II: An Experimental Investigation of Date-Initiation and Expectancy Violation." *Western Journal of Communication* 60 (1996): 195–213.

Mongeau, Paul, Colleen Carey, and M. Williams. "First Date Initiation and Enactment: An Expectancy Violation Perspective." In *Sex Differences and Similarities in Communication*, edited by Daniel Canary and K. Dindia, 413–26. Hillsdale, NJ: Lawrence Erlbaum Associates, 1998.

Mongeau, Paul, and Mary Clair Morr. "First Date Expectations." *Communication Research* 31 (2004): 3–35.

Moore, Monica. "Courtship Signaling and Adolescents: 'Girls Just Wanna Have Fun'?" *Journal of Sex Research* 32, no. 4 (1995): 319–28.

Muehlenhard, Charlene, and Carie Rodgers. "Token Resistance to Sex: New Perspectives on an Old Stereotype." In *Speaking of Sexuality*, edited by Kenneth Davidson and Nelwyn Moore, 280–89. Los Angeles, CA: Roxbury, 2005.

Murnen, Sarah, Perot Annette, and Donn Bryne. "Coping with Unwanted Sexual Activity: Normative Responses, Situational Determinants, and Individual Differences." *Journal of Sexual Research* 26 (1989): 85–106.

Nappi, Rossella E., Kathrin Wawra, and Sonja Schmitt. "Hypoactive Sexual Desire Disorder in Postmenopausal Women." *Gynecological Endocrinology* 22, no. 6 (2006): 318–23.

National Communication Association. *How Americans Communicate*. Washington, DC: National Communication Association, 2009.

National Communication Association. "Interview with Dr. Claude Miller." In *Communication Currents*, edited by Joanne Keyton, audiocast. Washington, DC: National Communication Association, 2009.

National Opinion Research Center. *GSS Report*. Edited by the University of Chicago. Chicago: University of Chicago, 2003.

Noar, Seth, Rick Zimmerman, and Katherine Atwood. "Safer Sex and Sexually Transmitted Infections from a Relationship Perspective." In *The Handbook of Sexuality in Close Relationships*, edited by John Harvey, Amy Wenzel, and Susan Sprecher, 519–44. Mahwah, NJ: Lawrence Erlbaum Associates, 2005.

Noland, Carey M. "Listening to the Sound of Silence: Gender Roles and Communication about Sex in Puerto Rico." *Sex Roles* 55, no. 5 (2006): 283–94.

Nolin, Mary J., and Karen K. Petersen. "Gender Differences in Parent-Child Communication about Sexuality: An Exploratory Study." *Journal of Adolescent Research* 7, no. 1 (1992): 59–79.

Papaharitou, Stamatis, Evangelia Nakopoulou, Martha Moraitou, Zoi Tsimt-
siou, Eleni Konstantinidou, and Dimitrios Hatzichristou. "Exploring
Sexual Attitudes of Students in Health Professions." *Journal of Sexual
Medicine* 5, no. 6 (2008): 1308–16.

Pardun, Carol J., Kelly Ladin L'Engle, and Jane D. Brown. "Linking Exposure
to Outcomes: Early Adolescents' Consumption of Sexual Content in Six
Media." *Mass Communication and Society* 8 (2005): 75–91.

Parrott, Roxanne, Ashley Duggan, and Veronica Duncan. "Promoting Patients' Full and Honest Disclosures during Conventions with Health
Caregivers." In *Balancing the Secrets of Private Disclosures*, edited by
Sandra Petronio, 137–49. Mahwah, NJ: Lawrence Erlbaum Associates,
2000.

Paul, Elizabeth L., and Kristen A. Hayes. "The Casualties of 'Casual' Sex: A
Qualitative Exploration of the Phenomenology of College Students'
Hookups." *Journal of Social and Personal Relationships* 19 (2002): 639–61.

Paul, Elizabeth L., Brian McManus, and Allison Hayes. "'Hookups': Characteristics and Correlates of College Students' Spontaneous and Anonymous Sexual Experiences." *Journal of Sex Research* 37 (2000): 76–88.

Peplau, Letitia Anne. "Human Sexuality: How Do Men and Women Differ?"
Current Directions in Psychological Science 12, no. 2 (2003): 37–40.

Peplau, Letitia Anne, and Linda D. Garnets. "A New Paradigm for Understanding Women's Sexuality and Sexual Orientation." *Journal of Social Issues* 56, no. 2 (2000): 329–50.

Perloff, Richard. *Persuading People to Have Safer Sex: Applications of Social Science
to the AIDS Crisis.* Mahwah, NJ: Lawrence Erlbaum Associates, 2001.

Petronio, Sandra. *Boundaries of Privacy: Dialectics of Disclosure.* Albany: State University of New York Press, 2002.

Phillips, Lynn M. *Flirting with Danger: Young Women's Reflections on Sexuality
and Domination.* New York: New York University Press, 2000.

Previti, Denise, and Paul R. Amato. "Is Infidelity a Cause or a Consequence of
Poor Marital Quality?" *Journal of Social and Personal Relationships* 21 (2004):
217–30.

Purnine, Daniel M., and Michael P. Carey. "Interpersonal Communication and
Sexual Adjustment: The Roles of Understanding and Agreement." *Journal of Consulting and Clinical Psychology* 65, no. 6 (1997): 1017–25.

Rabinowitz, Fredric E. "The Male-to-Male Embrace: Breaking the Touch Taboo
in a Men's Therapy Group." *Journal of Counseling and Development* 69,
no. 6 (1991): 574–76.

Rakel, Robert E. *Textbook of Family Practice.* 6th ed. Maryland Heights, MO:
MD Consult, 2002.

Regan, Pamela. *The Dating Game.* 2nd ed. Thousand Oaks, CA: Sage, 2008.

Regan, Pamela C., and Ellen Berscheid. "Gender Differences in Characteristics Desired in a Potential Sexual and Marriage Partner." *Journal of
Psychology and Human Sexuality* 9, no. 1 (1997): 25–37.

Regan, Paula. "Sex and the Attraction Process: Lessons from Science (and Shakespeare) on Lust, Love, Chastity, and Fidelity." In *The Handbook of Sexuality in Close Relationships*, edited by John Harvey, Amy Wenzel, and Susan Sprecher, 115–33. Mahwah, NJ: Lawrence Erlbaum Associates, 2004.

Ridely, Jane. "Gender and Couples: Do Men and Women Seek Different Kinds of Intimacy?" *Sexual and Marital Therapy* 8, no. 3 (1993): 243–53.

Rittenour, Christine E., and Melanie Booth-Butterfield. "College Students' Sexual Health: Investigating the Role of Peer Communication." *Qualitative Research Reports in Communication* 7 (2006): 57–65.

Roberts, Linda. "Fire and Ice in Marital Communication: Hostile and Distancing Behaviors as Predictors of Marital Distress." *Journal of Marriage and Family* 62, no. 3 (2000): 693–707.

Rose, Suzanna, and Irene H. Frieze. "Young Singles' Contemporary Dating Scripts." *Sex Roles* 28, no. 9 (1993): 499–509.

Rosen, Raymond C., and Stanley Althof. "Impact of Premature Ejaculation: The Psychological, Quality of Life, and Sexual Relationship Consequences." *Journal of Sexual Medicine* 5, no. 6 (2008): 1296–307.

Rosen, Raymond C., and Sandra R. Leiblum. "A Sexual Scripting Approach to Problems of Desire." In *Sexual Desire Disorders*, 168–91. New York: Guilford Press, 1988.

Rowland, David, Larry Crisler, and Donna Cox. "Flirting between College Students and Faculty." *Journal of Sex Research* 18, no. 4 (1982): 346–59.

Rubin, Alan M., Elizabeth M. Perse, and Robert A. Powell. "Loneliness, Parasocial Interaction and Local Television Viewing." *Human Communication Research* 12 (1985): 155–80.

Ryder, N., D. Ivens, and C. Sabin. "The Attitude of Patients towards Medical Students in a Sexual Health Clinic." *Sexually Transmitted Infections* 81, no. 5 (2005): 437–39.

Savin-Williams, Ritch. "Lesbian, Gay Male and Bisexual Adolescents." In *Lesbian, Gay, and Bisexual Identities over the Lifespan*, edited by Anthony D'Augelli and C.J. Patterson, 165–89. New York: Oxford University Press, 1996.

Schmitt, David. "Short and Long Term Mating Strategies: Additional Evolutionary Systems Relevant to Adolescent Sexuality." In *Romance and Sex in Adolescence and Emerging Adulthood: Risks and Opportunities*, edited by Ann C. Crouter and Alan Booth, 41–60. Mahwah, NJ: Lawrence Erlbaum Associates, 2006.

Schuster, M.A., R.M. Bell, L.P. Petersen, and D.E. Kanouse. "Communication between Adolescents and Physicians about Sexual Behavior and Risk Prevention." *Archives of Pediatrics and Adolescent Medicine* 150, no. 9 (1996): 906–13.

Schwartz, Pepper, Ann C. Crouter, and Alan Booth. "What Elicits Romance, Passion, and Attachment, and How Do They Affect Our Lives throughout the Life Cycle?" In *Romance and Sex in Adolescence and Emerging Adulthood: Risks and Opportunities*, edited by Ann C. Crouter and Alan Booth, 49–60. Mahwah, NJ: Lawrence Erlbaum Associates, 2006.

Segrin, C., and Robin Nabi. "Does Television Viewing Cultivate Unrealistic Expectations about Marriage?" *European Journal of Communication* 52 (2002): 247–63.

Segrin, Chris, and Mary Anne Fitzpatrick. "Depression and Verbal Aggressiveness in Different Marital Types." *Communication Studies* 43 (1992): 79–91.

Shotland, R. Lance, and Jane M. Craig. "Can Men and Women Differentiate between Friendly and Sexually Interested Behavior?" *Social Psychology Quarterly* 51, no. 1 (1988): 66–73.

Signorielli, Nancy. "Adolescents and Ambivalence toward Marriage: A Cultivation Analysis." *Youth and Society* 23, no. 1 (1991): 121–49.

Signorielli, Nancy. "Sex on Prime-Time in the 90's." *Communication Research Reports* 17, no. 1 (2000): 70–78.

Simon, William, and John Gagnon. "A Sexual Scripts Approach." In *Theories of Human Sexuality*, edited by J. H. Geer and W. O'Donahue, 363–83. New York: Plenum, 1987.

Simpson, Jeffry A., Steven W. Gangestad, and Michael Biek. "Personality and Nonverbal Social Behavior: An Ethological Perspective of Relationship Initiation." *Journal of Experimental Social Psychology* 29, no. 5 (1993): 434–61.

Smith, C. Veronica. "In Pursuit of 'Good' Sex: Self-Determination and the Sexual Experience." *Journal of Social and Personal Relationships* 24 (2007): 69–85.

Spitzberg, Brian H., and William R. Cupach, eds. *The Dark Side of Close Relationships*. Mahwah, NJ: Lawrence Erlbaum Associates, 1998.

Sprecher, Susan, and Diane Felmlee. "Insider Perspectives on Attraction." In *Handbook of Relationship Initiation*, edited by Susan Sprecher, Amy Wenzel, and John Harvey, 297–313. New York: Psychology Press, 2008.

Sprecher, Susan, Gardenia Harris, and Adena Meyers. "Perceptions of Sources of Sex Education and Targets of Sex Communication: Sociodemographic and Cohort Effects." *Journal of Sex Research* 45 (2008): 17–26.

Sprecher, Susan, and Kathleen McKinney. *Sexuality*. Newbury Park, CA: Sage, 1993.

Sprecher, Susan, and Pamela C. Regan. "Liking Some Things (in Some People) More Than Others: Partner Preferences in Romantic Relationships and Friendships." *Journal of Social and Personal Relationships* 19 (2002): 463–81.

Stauffer, John, and Richard Frost. "Male and Female Interest in Sexually-Oriented Magazines." *Journal of Communication* 26 (1976): 25–30.

Stepp, Laura Sessions. *Unhooked: How Young Women Pursue Sex, Delay Love, and Lose at Both*. New York: Riverhead Books, 2007.

Stewart, Stephanie, Heather Stinnett, and Lawrence B. Rosenfeld. "Sex Differences in Desired Characteristics of Short-Term and Long-Term Relationship Partners." *Journal of Social and Personal Relationships* 17 (2000): 843–53.

Tannen, Deborah. *You Just Don't Understand: Women and Men in Conversation.* New York: Morrow, 1990.

Tiefer, Leonore. "Sexual Behaviour and Its Medicalisation: Many (Especially Economic) Forces Promote Medicalisation." *British Medical Journal* 325, no. 7354 (2002): 896–900.

Tomlinson, J. "ABC of Sexual Health: Taking a Sexual History." *British Medical Journal* 317, no. 7172 (1998): 1573–76.

Trost, Melanie, and Jess Alberts. "An Evolutionary View on Understanding Sex Effects in Communicating Attraction." In *Sex Differences and Similarities in Communication: Critical Essays and Empirical Investigations of Sex and Gender in Interaction*, edited by Daniel Canary and Kathryn Dindia, 233–55. Mahwah, NJ: Lawrence Erlbaum Associates, 1998.

Waite, Linda J., and Kara Joyner. "Emotional Satisfaction and Physical Pleasure in Sexual Unions: Time Horizon, Sexual Behavior, and Sexual Exclusivity." *Journal of Marriage and Family* 63, no. 1 (2001): 247–64.

Walster, Elaine, William Walster, and Ellen Berscheid. *Equity: Theory and Research.* Boston: Allyn and Bacon, 1978.

Ward, L. Monique. "Talking about Sex: Common Themes about Sexuality in the Prime-Time Television Programs Children and Adolescents View Most." *Journal of Youth and Adolescence* 24, no. 5 (1995): 595–615.

Warszawski, J., and L. Meyer. "Sex Difference in Partner Notification: Results from Three Population Based Surveys in France." *Sexually Transmitted Infections* 78, no. 1 (2002): 45–49.

Watzlawick, Paul, Janet Beavin, and Don Jackson. *Pragmatics of Human Communication.* New York: W. W. Norton, 1967.

Welshimer, K. J., and S. E. Harris. "A Survey of Rural Parents' Attitudes toward Sexuality Education." *Journal of School Health* 64, no. 9 (1994): 347–52.

Widman, Laura, Deborah P. Welsh, James K. McNulty, and Katherine C. Little. "Sexual Communication and Contraceptive Use in Adolescent Dating Couples." *Journal of Adolescent Health* 39, no. 6 (2006): 893–99.

Wight, Daniel, Alison Parkes, Vicki Strange, Elizabeth Allen, Chris Bonell, and Marion Henderson. "The Quality of Young People's Heterosexual Relationships: A Longitudinal Analysis of Characteristics Shaping Subjective Experience." *Perspectives on Sexual and Reproductive Health* 40 (2008): 226–37.

Wolitski, Richard J., Bernard M. Branson, and Ann O'Leary. "'Gray Area Behaviors' and Partner Selection Strategies: Working toward a Comprehensive Approach to Reducing the Sexual Transmission of HIV." In *Beyond Condoms: Alternative Approaches to HIV Prevention*, 173–98. New York: Kluwer Academic/Plenum, 2002.

Wood, Julia. *But I Thought You Meant . . . Misunderstandings in Human Communication.* Mountain View, CA: Mayfield, 1998.

Wood, Julia. *Gendered Lives.* 7th ed. Belmont, CA: Thompson Wadsworth, 2007.

Wright, Kevin, Lisa Sparks, and Dan O'Hair. *Health Communication in the 21st Century.* Malden, MA: Blackwell, 2008.

Yelvington, Kevin. "Flirting in the Factory." *Journal of the Royal Anthropological Institute* 2 (1996): 313–33.

Young Pistella, Christine L., and Frank A. Bonati. "Adolescent Women's Recommendations for Enhanced Parent-Adolescent Communication about Sexual Behavior." *Child and Adolescent Social Work Journal* 16 (1999): 305–15.

Zillmann, D., and B.S. Sapolsky. "What Mediates the Effect of Mild Erotica on Annoyance and Hostile Behavior in Males?" *Journal of Personality and Social Psychology* 35, no. 8 (1977): 587–96.

Index

About the Author

DR. CAREY M. NOLAND is an award-winning author and professor who has over twenty years of experience teaching and researching in the area of sexual health communication. She has developed a unique approach to help people of all backgrounds overcome their fears and limitations regarding communication about sex. She has taught thousands of students and authored and produced over forty professional papers and publications on communication-related topics. Dr. Noland has traveled the world, from Southeast Asia to Latin America, teaching and studying communication.

In this book, Dr. Noland offers her readers an insightful understanding of communication with a dynamic and engaging writing style. She is a deeply committed advocate to helping people achieve healthy sexual relationships. She completed her undergraduate studies in economics and statistics from Boston University, while graduate work includes a Master's degree from the LBJ School of Public Affairs, University of Texas, Austin and a PhD in communication studies from Ohio University. She is currently an Associate Professor of Communication Studies at Northeastern University in Boston, MA.